Current Trends and Future Directions in Prosthetic and Implant Dentistry in the Digital Era

Current Trends and Future Directions in Prosthetic and Implant Dentistry in the Digital Era

Editors

Adolfo Di Fiore
Giulia Brunello

MDPI • Basel • Beijing • Wuhan • Barcelona • Belgrade • Manchester • Tokyo • Cluj • Tianjin

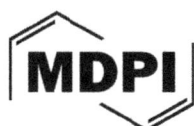

Editors
Adolfo Di Fiore
University of Padova
Italy

Giulia Brunello
University Hospital of Düsseldorf
Germany

Editorial Office
MDPI
St. Alban-Anlage 66
4052 Basel, Switzerland

This is a reprint of articles from the Special Issue published online in the open access journal *Journal of Clinical Medicine* (ISSN 2077-0383) (available at: https://www.mdpi.com/journal/jcm/special_issues/Prosthetic_and_Implant_Dentistry_in_the_Digital_Era).

For citation purposes, cite each article independently as indicated on the article page online and as indicated below:

LastName, A.A.; LastName, B.B.; LastName, C.C. Article Title. *Journal Name* **Year**, *Volume Number*, Page Range.

ISBN 978-3-0365-6049-6 (Hbk)
ISBN 978-3-0365-6050-2 (PDF)

© 2022 by the authors. Articles in this book are Open Access and distributed under the Creative Commons Attribution (CC BY) license, which allows users to download, copy and build upon published articles, as long as the author and publisher are properly credited, which ensures maximum dissemination and a wider impact of our publications.

The book as a whole is distributed by MDPI under the terms and conditions of the Creative Commons license CC BY-NC-ND.

Contents

Adolfo Di Fiore
Think Digital—The New Era in the Dentistry Field
Reprinted from: *J. Clin. Med.* **2022**, *11*, 4073, doi:10.3390/jcm11144073 . . . . **1**

Adolfo Di Fiore, Mattia Montagner, Stefano Sivolella, Edoardo Stellini, Burak Yilmaz and Giulia Brunello
Peri-Implant Bone Loss and Overload: A Systematic Review Focusing on Occlusal Analysis through Digital and Analogic Methods
Reprinted from: *J. Clin. Med.* **2022**, *11*, 4812, doi:10.3390/jcm11164812 . . . . **3**

Adolfo Di Fiore, Edoardo Stellini, Michele Basilicata, Patrizio Bollero and Carlo Monaco
Effect of Toothpaste on the Surface Roughness of the Resin-Contained CAD/CAM Dental Materials: A Systematic Review
Reprinted from: *J. Clin. Med.* **2022**, *11*, 767, doi:10.3390/jcm11030767 . . . . **17**

Diego Lops, Eugenio Romeo, Stefano Calza, Antonino Palazzolo, Lorenzo Viviani, Stefano Salgarello, Barbara Buffoli and Magda Mensi
Association between Peri-Implant Soft Tissue Health and Different Prosthetic Emergence Angles in Esthetic Areas: Digital Evaluation after 3 Years' Function
Reprinted from: *J. Clin. Med.* **2022**, *11*, 6243, doi:10.3390/jcm11216243 . . . . **27**

Jan van Hooft, Guido Kielenstijn, Jeroen Liebregts, Frank Baan, Gert Meijer, Jan D'haese, Ewald Bronkhorst and Luc Verhamme
Intraoral Scanning as an Alternative to Evaluate the Accuracy of Dental Implant Placements in Partially Edentate Situations: A Prospective Clinical Case Series
Reprinted from: *J. Clin. Med.* **2022**, *11*, 5876, doi:10.3390/jcm11195876 . . . . **39**

Vinicius Rizzo Marques, Gülce Çakmak, Hakan Yilmaz, Samir Abou-Ayash, Mustafa Borga Donmez and Burak Yilmaz
Effect of Scanned Area and Operator on the Accuracy of Dentate Arch Scans with a Single Implant
Reprinted from: *J. Clin. Med.* **2022**, *11*, 4125, doi:10.3390/jcm11144125 . . . . **53**

Maximiliane Amelie Schlenz, Julian Maximilian Stillersfeld, Bernd Wöstmann and Alexander Schmidt
Update on the Accuracy of Conventional and Digital Full-Arch Impressions of Partially Edentulous and Fully Dentate Jaws in Young and Elderly Subjects: A Clinical Trial
Reprinted from: *J. Clin. Med.* **2022**, *11*, 3723, doi:10.3390/jcm11133723 . . . . **65**

Gianmaria D'Addazio, Edit Xhajanka, Tonino Traini, Manlio Santilli, Imena Rexhepi, Giovanna Murmura, Sergio Caputi and Bruna Sinjari
Accuracy of DICOM–DICOM vs. DICOM–STL Protocols in Computer-Guided Surgery: A Human Clinical Study
Reprinted from: *J. Clin. Med.* **2022**, *11*, 2336, doi:10.3390/jcm11092336 . . . . **79**

Diego Lops, Eugenio Romeo, Michele Stocchero, Antonino Palazzolo, Barbara Manfredi and Luca Sbricoli
Marginal Bone Maintenance and Different Prosthetic Emergence Angles: A 3-Year Retrospective Study
Reprinted from: *J. Clin. Med.* **2022**, *11*, 2014, doi:10.3390/jcm11072014 . . . . **95**

Juan Ramón González Rueda, Irene García Ávila, Víctor Manuel de Paz Hermoso, Elena Riad Deglow, Álvaro Zubizarreta-Macho, Jesús Pato Mourelo, Javier Montero Martín and Sofía Hernández Montero
Accuracy of a Computer-Aided Dynamic Navigation System in the Placement of Zygomatic Dental Implants: An In Vitro Study
Reprinted from: *J. Clin. Med.* **2022**, *11*, 1436, doi:10.3390/jcm11051436 . . . . **105**

Giovanni Battista Menchini-Fabris, Paolo Toti, Roberto Crespi, Giovanni Crespi, Saverio Cosola and Ugo Covani
A Retrospective Digital Analysis of Contour Changing after Tooth Extraction with or without Using Less Traumatic Surgical Procedures
Reprinted from: *J. Clin. Med.* **2022**, *11*, 922, doi:10.3390/jcm11040922 . . . . **117**

Paolo Pesce, Francesco Bagnasco, Nicolò Pancini, Marco Colombo, Luigi Canullo, Francesco Pera, Eriberto Bressan, Marco Annunziata and Maria Menini
Trueness of Intraoral Scanners in Implant-Supported Rehabilitations: An In Vitro Analysis on the Effect of Operators' Experience and Implant Number
Reprinted from: *J. Clin. Med.* **2021**, *10*, 5917, doi:10.3390/jcm10245917 . . . . **133**

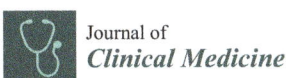

Editorial

Think Digital—The New Era in the Dentistry Field

Adolfo Di Fiore

Department of Neurosciences, Section of Prosthodontic and Digital Dentistry, School of Dentistry, University of Padova, 35122 Padova, Italy; adolfo.difiore@unipd.it

Citation: Di Fiore, A. Think Digital—The New Era in the Dentistry Field. *J. Clin. Med.* **2022**, *11*, 4073. https://doi.org/10.3390/jcm11144073

Received: 11 July 2022
Accepted: 13 July 2022
Published: 14 July 2022

Publisher's Note: MDPI stays neutral with regard to jurisdictional claims in published maps and institutional affiliations.

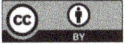

Copyright: © 2022 by the author. Licensee MDPI, Basel, Switzerland. This article is an open access article distributed under the terms and conditions of the Creative Commons Attribution (CC BY) license (https://creativecommons.org/licenses/by/4.0/).

In recent years the dental field has evolved incredibly due to the introduction of digital technology. Thanks to new devices such as intraoral and facial scanners, different clinical procedures have been facilitated by reducing clinical steps and operative time [1,2]. The most changes have emerged in the discipline of prosthetic dentistry, where advances in technology have provided the ability to realize a crown or an inlay in a few hours. However, such simplification is not of interest only to the daily clinic approach, but also to diagnosis, clinical training, and manufacturing methods. The three-dimensional environment allows clinicians and students to analyze bone quality and quantity, assess the tooth preparation, and to design a new smile. Moreover, the choice to realize types of dental prostheses with different techniques has opened a new scenario in dental materials science. New dental materials have been developed, improving the esthetics, and providing a better potential for long-term survival and stability. Although the development of material through subtractive manufacturing presents better mechanical and surface characteristics than additive manufacturing [3], the future will be additive. This manufacturing method is an eco-friendly technology, due to the lower environmental impact, the reduced waste of materials, and the use of recyclable materials. However, the question of whether digital dentistry is the past, present, or future remains without an answer. A unanimous consensus is not present among clinicians. Some prefer the use of a conventional workflow or use a combined workflow, whereas others apply a completely digital workflow. The reasons are several, but I think that this difference is mainly attributable to the reluctance of clinicians to change their daily workflow. Where the conventional workflow results in the omission of some preparation errors, the digital workflow does not. All clinical steps must be executed with the utmost accuracy. For example, the incorrect management of an interim crown does not allow the control of many problems associated with digital impressions, such as localized bleeding, the retraction technique, and the limits of scanners to acquire the subgingival vertical finish line. Indeed, only high-quality dentistry can take advantage of digital dentistry, more so than poor-quality dentistry. It is fundamental to remember that the patient is the most important person in dental treatment, and therefore, must be the first person that benefits from digital dental procedures. For all clinicians and students, I give one suggestion: think digital for better daily dentistry.

Funding: This research received no external funding.

Conflicts of Interest: The authors declare no conflict of interest.

References

1. Di Fiore, A.; Vigolo, P.; Graiff, L.; Stellini, E. Digital vs Conventional Workflow for Screw-Retained Single-Implant Crowns: A Comparison of Key Considerations. *Int. J. Prosthodont.* **2018**, *31*, 577–579. [CrossRef] [PubMed]
2. Di Fiore, A.; Meneghello, R.; Graiff, L.; Savio, G.; Vigolo, P.; Monaco, C.; Stellini, E. Full arch digital scanning systems performances for implant-supported fixed dental prostheses: A comparative study of 8 intraoral scanners. *J. Prosthodont. Res.* **2019**, *63*, 396–403. [CrossRef] [PubMed]
3. Di Fiore, A.; Meneghello, R.; Brun, P.; Rosso, S.; Gattazzo, A.; Stellini, E.; Yilmaz, B. Comparison of the flexural and surface properties of milled, 3D-printed, and heat polymerized PMMA resins for denture bases: An in vitro study. *J. Prosthodont. Res.* **2021**. [CrossRef] [PubMed]

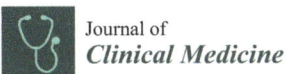

Review

Peri-Implant Bone Loss and Overload: A Systematic Review Focusing on Occlusal Analysis through Digital and Analogic Methods

Adolfo Di Fiore [1,*], Mattia Montagner [2], Stefano Sivolella [1], Edoardo Stellini [1], Burak Yilmaz [3,4,5] and Giulia Brunello [1,6]

1. Department of Neurosciences, School of Dentistry, University of Padova, 35128 Padova, Italy
2. Private Practice, 35121 Padova, Italy
3. Department of Reconstructive Dentistry and Gerodontology, School of Dental Medicine, University of Bern, 3012 Bern, Switzerland
4. Department of Restorative, Preventive and Pediatric Dentistry, School of Dental Medicine, University of Bern, 3012 Bern, Switzerland
5. Division of Restorative and Prosthetic Dentistry, The Ohio State University, Columbus, OH 43210, USA
6. Department of Oral Surgery, University Hospital Düsseldorf, 40225 Düsseldorf, Germany
* Correspondence: adolfo.difiore@unipd.it

Abstract: The present review aimed to assess the possible relationship between occlusal overload and peri-implant bone loss. In accordance with the PRISMA guidelines, the MEDLINE, Scopus, and Cochrane databases were searched from January 1985 up to and including December 2021. The search strategy applied was: (dental OR oral) AND implants AND (overload OR excessive load OR occlusal wear) AND (bone loss OR peri-implantitis OR failure). Clinical studies that reported quantitative analysis of occlusal loads through digital contacts and/or occlusal wear were included. The studies were screened for eligibility by two independent reviewers. The quality of the included studies was assessed using the Risk of Bias in Non-randomized Studies of Interventions (ROBINS-I) tool. In total, 492 studies were identified in the search during the initial screening. Of those, 84 were subjected to full-text evaluation, and 7 fulfilled the inclusion criteria (4 cohort studies, 2 cross-sectional, and 1 case-control). Only one study used a digital device to assess excessive occlusal forces. Four out of seven studies reported a positive correlation between the overload and the crestal bone loss. All of the included studies had moderate to serious overall risk of bias, according to the ROBINS-I tool. In conclusion, the reported data relating the occlusal analysis to the peri-implant bone level seem to reveal an association, which must be further investigated using new digital tools that can help to standardize the methodology.

Keywords: dental implant; occlusion; overloading; complications; implant-supported restorations; marginal bone loss

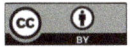

1. Introduction

Implant dentistry represents a safe and predictable treatment modality to rehabilitate both complete and partially edentulous patients [1]. The number of dental implants fitted every year is increasing; in the US, their prevalence rose from 0.7% in 1999 to 5.7% in 2015, with a projection of 23% in 2026 [1]. This tendency can be ascribed to an increase in oral-health-related quality of life [2,3]. In a recent systematic review, which included longitudinal studies with a follow-up of at least 10 years for a total of 7711 implants, a cumulative mean survival rate of 94.6% (SD 5.97%) was reported, with variation from 73.4% to 100% [4].

Several factors are reported to be associated with crestal bone loss (CBL), including bacterial colonization and the presence of a micro-gap between abutment and implant [5,6]. Contradictory findings on the role of occlusal overload on peri-implant bone loss have been reported, with limited evidence supporting the cause-and-effect relationship [7]. Overload is generally considered to be an excessive occlusal load on the implant-supported fixed dental prosthesis (FDP), leading to high stress on the peri-implant bone tissue [8–10]. An imbalance in the occlusal load may generate stress at the bone–implant coronal first contact point [11], which might increase the incidence of CBL [12].

The potential detrimental effect of overload in implant therapy was first observed by Adell [13] in 1981. Quirynen et al. [14] examined the effect of overload, finding an excessive CBL in the first year of load in patients who were rehabilitated using implant-supported prosthesis in both jaws and who presented a lack of anterior guidance or parafunctional activity. Naert et al. [15] also reported similar results under the same conditions. In more recent studies [16,17], which either analyze the characteristics of early and late implant failure or assess implant survival rates in bone of different qualities, implants failed due to more marked occlusal areas identified through articulating paper. However, many reviews reported a lack of evidence regarding the positive correlation between the overload and the CBL [7,18–21]. These heterogenous results may be attributable to the different methods of analyzing the overload. Clinical studies have assessed the presence of overload in relation to the length of cantilever, bruxism, tooth clenching, or the presence of an implant-supported prosthesis as the antagonist [18–21]; however, the results are difficult to compare and repeat. With the development of digital technology, some devices have been introduced in the dental market to assess occlusal force, but few are discussed in the articles published in the literature [22–24]. However, almost all of the articles concluded that using digital technology allows for more accurate constructions and the more precise balancing of occlusal relationships [22–24].

Contradictory results were found in animal studies. Some authors reported increased marginal bone loss [25], a loss of osseointegration [26], or crater-like bone resorption [27] in the presence of overload. However, excessive loading did not result in any difference in histologically assessed peri-implant bone loss, either in healthy implants nor in implants affected by ligature-induced peri-implantitis in primates [28]. In another study in dogs, no difference was reported in terms of the loss of osseointegration or marginal bone loss between non-loaded implants and implants subjected to excessive occlusal load after eight months [29]. In an animal study where a lateral load was applied to implants for 24 weeks, a structural adaptation of the peri-implant bone was histologically observed in the test implants compared to unloaded controls, in terms of higher bone density and mineralized bone-to-implant contact [30].

Overload potentially plays a role in the behavior of peri-implant bone; however, its role in the onset and progression of bone loss is still unclear. Therefore, a systematic review is needed to give a clear idea of the problem. This uncertainty has also been attributed to the difficulties in measuring the magnitude and the direction of forces in clinical studies [7]. The heterogeneity of the data regarding this subject perpetuates doubts among researchers and clinicians. Furthermore, to the best of the authors' knowledge, there is no previous review on the topic focusing only on the utilization of repeatable and quantifiable overload assessment methods. Therefore, due to the lack of clear results, this systematic review aimed to assess the possible relationship between overload, assessed through digital occlusal analysis and/or occlusal wear, and crestal bone loss.

2. Materials and Methods

To investigate the possible correlation between overload and crestal bone loss (CBL), an extensive search was conducted to identify scientific studies focused on the problem. This systematic review was conducted in accordance with the Preferred Reporting Items for Systematic Reviews (PRISMA) 2020 statement [31]. The protocol for this review was registered with the international prospective register of systematic reviews (PROSPERO) with registration no. CRD42021250518. The clinical question was formulated using the PICO strategy (population: patients with an osseointegrated implant; intervention: implant occlusal overload; comparison: absence of implant occlusal overloading; outcome:

crestal bone loss). The PICO question was structured as follows: "Does implant occlusal overloading influence crestal bone loss around osseointegrated dental implants?".

2.1. Search Strategy

A broad electronic search for relevant publications, published from 1 January 1985 to 31 December 2021, was performed across MEDLINE (via PubMed), the Cochrane Central Register of Controlled Trials (CENTRAL), and Scopus. The electronic search strategy applied was: (dental or oral) AND implants AND (overload OR excessive load OR occlusal wear) AND (bone loss OR peri-implantitis OR failure). No language restrictions were applied. To identify other eligible studies, a manual search based on the reference lists of the most relevant systematic reviews on the topic, and of all the articles retrieved from the electronic databases, was conducted.

2.2. Inclusion and Exclusion Criteria

The following criteria had to be met for inclusion: clinical human studies, including randomized controlled trials (RCTs), cohort prospective or retrospective studies, case-control studies, and cross-sectional studies, which evaluated bone loss around osseointegrated dental implants subjected to overload (assessed through digital occlusal analysis and/or occlusal wear) with a follow-up of one or more years after prosthetic loading [17,19]. The following were excluded: animal studies, case reports, case series, guidelines, reviews, and in silico (3D element finite analysis) and in vitro studies. Clinical studies assessing the presence of overload by the length of cantilever, bruxism, tooth clenching, or the presence of an implant-supported prosthesis as an antagonist were also excluded due to the impossibility of comparing the data.

2.3. Study Selection and Data Extraction

The published articles were first screened by one reviewer (M.M.), by title and abstract. In the second step, the full texts of the selected articles were evaluated by two independent reviewers (A.D.F. and M.M.). The agreement between the two reviewers was assessed by means of the Cohen's Kappa coefficient. Disagreements were resolved by discussion between the authors. The following data were extracted: title, authors, year of publication, journal in which the research was published, study design, number of patients and implants, patient characteristics, implant characteristics, type of prosthesis, follow-up, assessment methods (occlusal wear assessment), and main results. To simplify the terminology, all the terms used in the literature to identify the radiographic changes of peri-implant bone over time (e.g., crestal bone level, marginal bone level, crestal bone loss, marginal bone loss) were combined under the acronym CBL (crestal bone loss) and used as synonyms throughout this systematic review. Data were sought to find a difference in mean CBL (in mm) between overloaded and non-overloaded implants. Authors were contacted in order to acquire missing information, when necessary.

2.4. Quality Assessment

The quality of each included study was individually assessed. In accordance with the Cochrane Collaboration guidelines, the Risk of Bias in Non-randomized Studies of Interventions (ROBINS-I) tool was utilized [32]. Using this tool, seven domains (i.e., confounding, selection, classification of interventions, deviations from the intended intervention, missing data, measurement of outcomes, and reporting results) for each included study were classified at "low", "moderate", "serious", or "critical" risk of bias. Then, an overall score was given, judging the study at "low risk of bias" when it was assessed "low" in all domains, at "moderate risk of bias" when it was assessed "low" or "moderate" in all domains, at "serious risk of bias" when it was assessed "serious" in at least one domain, or at "critical risk of bias" when it was assessed "critical" in at least one domain.

3. Results

The flow diagram of the search results is presented in Figure 1.

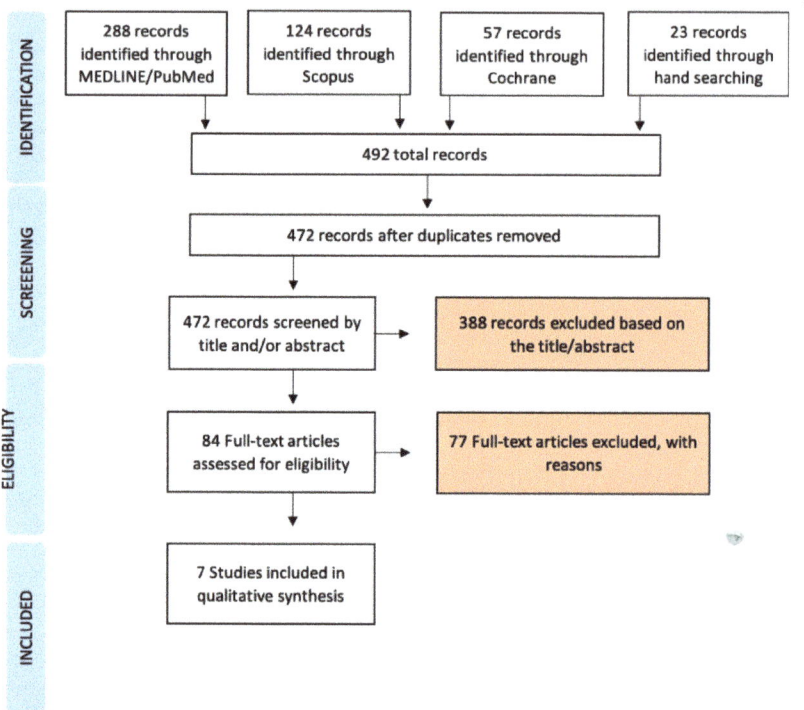

Figure 1. PRISMA flow chart of articles screened, withdrawn, and included in the review process.

The electronic search produced a total of 469 potentially relevant publications. Then, 23 additional records were found through a manual search, yielding a total of 492 studies. After the removal of duplicated studies, 472 records were obtained, of which 388 were excluded after title and abstract screening. After full-text evaluation of 84 records, only seven articles fulfilled the inclusion criteria and were included for qualitative analysis. The main reasons for exclusion were: animal research (n = 21) [25–30,33–46], reviews (n = 26) [6,7,9,12,14,18–20,47–64], in silico (n = 11) [65–75], in vitro (n = 3) [76–78], guidelines (n = 3) [21,79,80], case reports (n = 6) [10,81–85], lack of occlusal assessment (n = 1) [86], overload assessment method (n = 6), i.e., by maximum bite force [87], or bruxism habits [88–90], or length of cantilever [91], or type of antagonist [15].

The kappa values for inter-reviewer agreement for full-text selection was 0.89, indicating high agreement between the reviewers. Of the seven included articles, four were cohort studies [92–95], two were cross-sectional studies [96,97], and one was a case-control study [98]. No RCT was found to be eligible. Details of the included studies are reported in Table 1.

Table 1. Main features of the included studies.

Author(s), Year	Study Design	Total No. of Patients	Total No. of Implants	No. of Compromized Implants	Implant Diameter and Length [mm] §	Other Implant Features *	Type of Prosthesis	Follow-up (Range or ±SD) [Years] °	Occlusal Analysis	Correlation Overload–Cretal Bone Loss (Y/N)
Canullo et al., 2016 [98]	Retrospective case-control study	56	332	125	D < 4: 26 D = 4: 279 D > 4: 27 L not reported	Peri-implantitis group: Rough (n = 85) Smooth (n = 40)	Healthy implant group: Screwed (n = 127) Cemented (n = 80) Peri-implantitis group: Screwed (n = 64) Cemented (n = 61)	Healthy implant group: 6.48 ± 3.57 Peri-implantitis group: 5.94 ± 3.16	Fracture or chipping of the veneering; loss of retention; dynamic occlusal measurement by T-Scan III; occlusal photographs	Y**
Carlsson et al., 2000 [94]	Prospective cohort study	47 (of which 13 received treatment in both jaws)	343 (273 mandible; 75 maxilla)	8 (7 before loading)	D not reported L = 10 mm	Standard Brånemark implants (Nobel Biocare)	Full-arch implant-supported FDP (resin teeth)	15 (mandibular implants) 10.5 (8 to 13; maxillary implants)	Occlusal wear; bite force	N
Dalago et al., 2017 [96]	Retrospective cross-sectional study	183	938	89 (16 lost; 6 inactivated; 67 peri-implantitis)	D < 3.5 (n = 148) D = 3.5 (n = 575) D > 3.5 (n = 193) L < 9 (n = 796) L ≥ 9 (n = 120)	Connection: External Hexagon (n = 400) Internal Hexagon (n = 516)	Fixed restoration: Screwed (n = 436) Cemented (n = 480) Type of prosthesis: Single (n = 167) Partial (n = 522) Total (n = 227)	Mean: 5.64 (range 1 to 14)	Coronal fracture; wear facets	Y**
Engel et al., 2001 [95]	Prospective cohort study	379	379	21	D = 3.5 (n = 44) D = 3.5-4 (n = 153) D = 4.5-7 (n = 182) L not reported	Frialit-2 (n = 227) Bonefit (n = 51) IMZ (n = 47) Tübingen (n = 47) Brånemark (n = 6) TPS (n = 1)	Type of prostheses: Single (n = 188) Partial (n = 84) Overdenture (n = 107) Occlusal material: Ceramic (n = 182) Non-ceramic (n = 197)	Mean: 6 (range 1 to 10)	Wear facets	N
Lindquist et al., 1988 [92]	Prospective cohort study	46 25 (group 1) 21 (group 2)	276	N/A	Not reported	Brånemark implants	Mandibular full-arch implant-supported FDP	Group 1: 5½ to 6 Group 2: 3 to 4	Bite force; attrition and occlusal wear	Y

Table 1. Cont.

Author(s), Year	Study Design	Total No. of Patients	Total No. of Implants	No. of Compromized Implants	Implant Diameter and Length [mm] §	Other Implant Features *	Type of Prosthesis	Follow-up (Range or ±SD) [Years] °	Occlusal Analysis	Correlation Overload–Crestal Bone Loss (Y/N) **
Lindquist et al., 1996 [93]	Prospective cohort study	47 26 (group 1) 21 (group 2)	273	3	Not reported	Brånemark implants	Mandibular full-arch implant-supported FDP Mean cantilever length left = 14.7 mm (7 to 20) Mean cantilever length right= 15 mm (7 to 20)	Group 1: 15 Group 2: 10	Bite force; attrition and occlusal wear	N
Kissa et al., 2020 [97]	Retrospective cross-sectional study	145	642	146	Not reported	SA (n = 221) SLA (n = 161) HA (n = 260)	Fixed restoration: Screwed (n = 436) Cemented (n = 480)	Mean: 6.4 (1 to 16) (1 to 3: 242) (4 to 8: 226) (>8: 174)	Occlusal wear	Y

§ No. of implants per type reported into brackets; * Roughness; connection etc.; ** correlation with peri-implantitis, which according to the provided definition includes CBL; ° based on implant age; D, implant diameter; FDP: fixed dental prosthesis; HA, hydroxylapatite particle-blasted and acid-washed surface; L: implant length; SA, sandblasted and acid-etched surface; SLA, sandblasted with large grit and acid-etched surface; TPS, titanium plasma-spray.

Four studies [92,96–98] found a positive correlation between overload and CBL, while in the other three [93–95] no correlation was found. In two studies [96,98], a correlation was found between overload and peri-implantitis, which includes the radiographic detection of peri-implant bone loss as assessed according to the provided definition. Specifically, the case control study of Canullo et al. [98] identified the presence of overload with OR [95% CI] = 18.70 [5.5–63.2] ($p < 0.001$) as a predictor of peri-implantitis. Furthermore, Dalago et al. [96] found a positive relationship between peri-implantitis and prosthetic wear facets on crown and dentures in the univariate and in the multi-factor analysis (OR [95% CI] = 2.4 [1.2–4.8] $p = 0.032$). Kissa [97] reported higher probing depth and CBL in patients with facets on two or more posterior teeth. For Lindquist et al. [92], the length of the cantilever extensions and occlusal wear tended to be two factors implicated in increased CBL around the mesial implants. Indeed, the authors demonstrated a correlation between occlusal wear and CBL [92]. Conflicting results were reported in remaining three studies [93–95], which concluded that occlusal wear did not affect the annual vertical bone loss rate. The risk of bias in the seven studies included was assessed, and is summarized in Table 2.

Table 2. Risk of bias assessment (ROBINS-I) L = "low risk of bias"; M = "moderate risk of bias"; S = "serious risk of bias"; C = "critical risk of bias".

Study	Pre-Intervention		At Intervention	Post-Intervention				Overall Risk of Bias
	Confounding	Selection	Classification of Intervention	Deviation from Intended Intervention	Missing Data	Measurement of Outcome	Reporting Result	
Canullo et al., 2016 [98]	L	M	L	N/A	L	L	L	M
Carlsson et al., 2000 [94]	L	L	M	N/A	L	M	S	S
Dalago et al., 2017 [96]	L	M	M	N/A	L	L	L	M
Engel et al., 2001 [95]	L	L	M	N/A	S	M	M	S
Lindquist et al., 1988 [92]	L	L	M	N/A	L	M	S	S

N/A: not applicable.

All of the included studies had moderate to serious overall risk of bias. Specifically, all of the studies investigated possible confounding factors. Three studies [96–98] were deemed to have "moderate risk of bias" for the selection of participants, due to their retrospective design. All of the studies except one [98] presented a "moderate risk of bias" for classification of intervention, because the overload presence was identified by occlusal wear. Engel et al. [95] had a follow-up rate < 80% and no description of patients lost, hence it had a severe risk of bias in missing data. None of the four cohort studies [92–95] had an independent blind assessment of the outcomes. Only three studies [96–98] reported a complete data set of the results.

4. Discussion

This systematic review aimed to collect articles related to the relationship between overload and CBL. Only seven clinical studies were included; four showed a correlation between overload and CBL [92,96–98]. The main problem in this field of investigation is the proper assessment of the presence of overload and the quantification of its value; indeed, it is clinically difficult to measure occlusal forces during natural functioning [60]. Several methods have been proposed to detect excessive force on implant-supported fixed dental prostheses (FDPs), such as occlusal wear or wear facets, bruxism, reported tooth clenching, maximum bite force, the type of antagonist, and the length of the cantilever [52]. However, none of these signs are pathognomonic of the presence of overload, and they cannot provide a reproducible, quantifiable, absolute, or relative value.

Lindquist et al. [92] evaluated factors related to CBL in 276 dental implants in 46 patients, divided in two groups by follow-up time (Group 1: 3–4 years; group 2: 5–6 years). The authors found that in group 1, the mean bone loss was positively correlated ($p < 0.05$) to the length of the cantilever extension. In group 2, the correlations were similar, but they did not reach a statistically significant level. After six years, seven patients with long cantilevers (length = 15 mm) had a mean loss of 0.95 mm around the mesial implant, whereas six patients with short cantilevers (length < 15 mm) had a loss of 0.61 mm. The presence of load in long cantilevers seems to generate higher forces on the mesial implant than on the posterior ones, like a lever creating tensile forces on medial implant. However, subsequent studies did not find any correlation between CBL and short cantilevers [93,94] or long cantilevers [15,91]. In group 2, clenching and recorded occlusal wear were found to be correlated with CBL with Spearman's rank correlation coefficients of 0.41 ($0.01 < p < 0.05$) and 0.46, respectively ($0.01 < p < 0.05$). The same sample of patients was re-evaluated [93] for 12 to 15 years. According to the new statistical analysis, the factors related to CBL were poor oral hygiene, smoking, and anterior position of implants. Contrary to previous analysis, occlusal wear, the length of the cantilever, and reported tooth clenching did not present any significant correlation with CBL in the long-term follow-up. Carlsson et al. [94] conducted a cohort clinical study, with a follow-up of 15 years, on 47 edentulous patients rehabilitated with a mandibular complete-arch implant-supported FDP. During clinical examinations, 13 of the 47 patients received a maxillary complete-arch implant-supported FDP, whereas the other 34 had a removable complete denture as the antagonist. This study failed to find any correlation between occlusal wear and CBL. Similar results regarding the CBL in lower implants were recorded in patients with a complete-arch implant-supported FDP as the antagonist, as well as in those with a complete maxillary denture. This finding is in conflict with the observations of Quirynen et al. [15] and Naert et al. [88], who found a relation between CBL and the presence of an implant-supported FDP as the antagonist. The three studies discussed above were performed by one group of researchers, who followed the same selection criteria, treatment principles, and examination procedures [92–94]. The authors reported 11 implant losses in a total of 619 inserted implants, with 9 of the losses occurring before loading. The mean CBL was 0.9 mm both in the first sample of patients [92–94] and in the second one [94].

In the study of Engel et al. [95], all implant-supported FDPs presenting a shiny flat area or a flattening of the cusp tips were reported as wear facets. In this longitudinal study that evaluated implant-supported FDPs and overdentures on 379 patients, no correlation between occlusal wear and CBL was observed. However, occlusal wear was rare in implant-supported FDPs (14%) and more common in overdentures (43%) [99–101]. Among the studies included in the present review, only Engel et al. [95] investigated the influence of overload on peri-implant bone levels in the presence of different types of prostheses (i.e., overdentures, fixed partial prostheses, and single crowns), reporting no significant correlation.

In a cross-sectional study of 938 implants with different follow-up times (1 to 14 years, mean = 5.64 years), Dalago et al. [96] found a prevalence of 7.3% for peri-implantitis. In the univariate analysis, wear facets on the prosthetic crown were positively associated with peri-implantitis, and the same correlation was demonstrated in the multi-factor analysis with OR [95% CI] = 2.4 [1.2–4.8] ($p = 0.032$). Similar findings in another cross-sectional study on 642 implants were reported by Kissa et al. [97]. In the univariate analysis in patients with occlusal wear on the posterior teeth, the mean probing depth (PD) of the implants was 5.69 mm and mean implant CBL was 2.26 mm, while in patients without posterior occlusal wear, these values were 4.77 mm ($p = 0.004$) and 1.85 mm ($p = 0.02$), respectively. In the multivariate analysis, the mean PD in patients with posterior occlusal wear was 5.94, while this value was 4.96 mm in patients without posterior occlusal wear ($p = 0.01$). In the multivariate analysis, mean CBL and wear facets did not reach a significant correlation ($p = 0.2$); however, a trend of higher CBL was observed in patients with wear facets (mean = 2.91 mm) than in those without wear facets (mean = 2.69 mm). Thus, the wear of a prosthesis can be considered a sign of occlusal dysfunction, and may be associated with the presence of overload. However, the identification of wear facets does not allow for the measurement of the magnitude and direction of the forces.

Digital technologies are opening new possibilities for occlusal contact registration. In the retrospective case-control study carried out by Canullo et al. [98], static and dynamic contacts were recorded using a digital occlusal analysis device. The authors included only patients with at least two implants, with one or more affected by peri-implantitis. They assigned the implants affected by peri-implantitis (125) to the case group and the healthy implants (207) to the control group. Overload was reported in 3 implants in the healthy group and in 27 implants in the peri-implantitis group, with OR [95% CI] = 18.70 [5.5–63.2] (p = 0.0001). Therefore, excessive forces in an unbalanced occlusion were identified as the predictor of peri-implantitis. However, an accuracy of 82.35% and the small sample size were indicated as the limitations of the study by the authors. The combination of inadequate oral hygiene and signs of elevated occlusal load was found to have an impact on bone resorption [92], as well as on probing depth [97]. Moreover, other tools, such as the use of photoactivated blue-O toluidine [102], could be helpful in identifying peri-implantitis and preventing the development of the disease.

These findings are in agreement with those reported in other reviews [52,55,62] and in an animal study in monkey mandibles [37].

Contradictory results on the effects of overload on dental implants have also been found among animal studies. However, it has been frequently reported that overloaded implants exhibit higher bone–implant contact than unloaded implants [33,46]. This can be investigated only in animal models, owing to the possibility of sacrificing the animals and performing histological assessments of the peri-implant tissues. Therefore, load on implants seems to favor the quality of the peri-implant bone and enhance the osseointegration up to certain limits of load [103]. Above these values, the positive bone remodeling may involve a loss of osseointegration, mostly in presence of high lateral and dynamic forces [35,43]. Finally, in an animal model, peri-implant bone subjected to overload exhibited characteristic histological features. Unlike the implants affected by plaque-induced peri-implantitis, overloaded implants, which were losing osteointegration, presented a fibrous tissue between the bone and the implant surface, with a negligible inflammatory infiltrate in peri-implant soft tissues [49].

In summary, the main limitation encountered in the majority of the included studies, and in this field of research in general, arises from the utilization of assessment methods that are neither repeatable nor quantifiable. The absence of universally recognized threshold force values for the definition of overload is also a limitation for research studies on this topic. In the only included study that utilized a digital tool for assessing occlusal loading [98], overload was defined as an intensive red point resulting from the digital occlusal analysis system. The absence of a threshold value to use as a reference for digital occlusal checks in future research constitutes a limitation of the present review. Digital tools might represent a valid solution to overcome the limitations of traditional methods for the registration of occlusal contacts and the collection of quantitative data. These devices allow for the recording of occlusal forces, and for the intensity and presence of overload to be identified. Moreover, it is possible to convert the occlusal load into a numeric value that can be compared and analyzed. However, such tools are expensive. Conventional methods, such as articulating papers, impression waxes, and shim-stock foils, might be considered less reliable and objective as compared to digital tools [103]. Other limitations can be attributed to the restricted use of keywords during the electronic search strategy, which was complemented by an extensive manual search. However, the inclusion criteria would still have limited the results obtained. Finally, all the included studies presented a moderate to serious overall risk of bias.

5. Conclusions

Large clinical trials with long term follow-ups, which use repeatable and quantifiable assessment methods, are needed to clarify the role of overload on peri-implant bone loss. There is a need to identify a threshold value of overload that is able to trigger peri-implant bone loss. The use of standardized parameters would also allow for comparison among different clinical studies. The influence of implant features (e.g., design, connection, surface topography, diameter), restorative materials, and the type of implant-supported restorations in the onset and progression of overload-triggered peri-implant bone loss should be further explored. In this context, finite element analysis (FEA) may also contribute to a better definition of the influence of loading variation. For instance, FEA has been applied to investigate the influence on stress of the prosthetic designs associated with implants of varying lengths and distribution [104], of the prosthetic screw design [105], or of the distribution of occlusal contacts [106]. Another area that should be investigated concerns the extent to which the resolution of occlusal overload could be effective in limiting the progression of prosthetically triggered peri-implant bone loss. In the present review, the reported data relating the occlusal analysis to peri-implant bone level seem to reveal an association; this association must be further investigated using new digital tools that can help to standardize the methodology.

Author Contributions: Conceptualization, A.D.F. and G.B.; methodology, S.S.; validation, M.M., A.D.F. and G.B.; formal analysis, M.M.; investigation, S.S.; data curation, B.Y.; writing—original draft preparation, A.D.F.; writing—review and editing, G.B.; visualization, E.S.; supervision, E.S. All authors have read and agreed to the published version of the manuscript.

Funding: This research received no external funding.

Institutional Review Board Statement: Not applicable.

Informed Consent Statement: Not applicable.

Data Availability Statement: Not applicable.

Conflicts of Interest: The authors declare no conflict of interest.

References

1. Elani, H.W.; Starr, J.R.; Da Silva, J.D.; Gallucci, G.O. Trends in Dental Implant Use in the U.S., 1999–2016, and Projections to 2026. *J. Dent. Res.* **2018**, *97*, 1424–1430. [CrossRef] [PubMed]
2. Wang, Y.; Bäumer, D.; Ozga, A.K.; Körner, G.; Bäumer, A. Patient satisfaction and oral health-related quality of life 10 years after implant placement. *BMC Oral Health* **2021**, *21*, 30. [CrossRef]
3. Perea, C.; Del Río, J.; Preciado, A.; Lynch, C.D.; Celemín, A.; Castillo-Oyagüe, R. Validation of the 'Quality of Life with Implant Prostheses (QoLIP-10)' questionnaire for wearers of cement-retained implant-supported restorations. *J. Dent.* **2015**, *43*, 1021–1031. [CrossRef] [PubMed]
4. Moraschini, V.; Poubel, L.A.D.C.; Ferreira, V.F.; Barboza, E.D.S.P. Evaluation of survival and success rates of dental implants reported in longitudinal studies with a follow-up period of at least 10 years: A systematic review. *Int. J. Oral Maxillofac. Surg.* **2015**, *44*, 377–388. [CrossRef] [PubMed]
5. Zheng, Z.; Ao, X.; Xie, P.; Jiang, F.; Chen, W. The biological width around implant. *J. Prosthodont. Res.* **2021**, *65*, 11–18. [CrossRef]
6. Oh, T.-J.; Yoon, J.; Misch, C.E.; Wang, H.-L. The Causes of Early Implant Bone Loss: Myth or Science? *J. Periodontol.* **2002**, *73*, 322–333. [CrossRef]
7. Bertolini, M.M.; Del Bel Cury, A.A.; Pizzoloto, L.; Acapa, I.R.H.; Shibli, J.A.; Bordin, D. Does traumatic occlusal forces lead to peri-implant bone loss? A systematic review. *Braz. Oral Res.* **2019**, *33*, e069. [CrossRef]
8. Uribe, R.; Peñarrocha, M.; Sanchis, J.M.; García, O. Marginal peri-implantitis due to occlusal overload. A case report. *Med. Oral* **2004**, *9*, 160–162.
9. Graves, C.V.; Harrel, S.K.; Rossmann, J.A.; Kerns, D.; Gonzalez, J.A.; Kontogiorgos, E.D.; Al-Hashimi, I.; Abraham, C. The Role of Occlusion in the Dental Implant and Peri-implant Condition: A Review. *Open Dent. J.* **2016**, *10*, 594–601. [CrossRef]
10. Merin, R.L. Repair of peri-implant bone loss after occlusal adjustment: A case report. *J. Am. Dent. Assoc.* **2014**, *145*, 1058–1062. [CrossRef]
11. Rangert, B.; Jemt, T.; Jörneus, L. Forces and moments on Branemark implants. *Int. J. Oral Maxillofac. Implant.* **1989**, *4*, 241–247.
12. Misch, C.E.; Suzuki, J.B.; Misch-Dietsh, F.M.; Bidez, M.W. A positive correlation between occlusal trauma and peri-implant bone loss: Literature support. *Implant Dent.* **2005**, *14*, 108–116. [CrossRef] [PubMed]

13. Adell, R.; Lekholm, U.; Rockler, B.; Brånemark, P.-I. A 15-year study of osseointegrated implants in the treatment of the edentulous jaw. *Int. J. Oral Surg.* **1981**, *10*, 387–416. [CrossRef]
14. Van Steenberghe, D.; Naert, I.; Jacobs, R.; Quirynen, M. Influence of inflammatory reactions vs. occlusal loading on peri-implant marginal bone level. *Adv. Dent. Res.* **1999**, *13*, 130–135. [CrossRef] [PubMed]
15. Quirynen, M.; Naert, I.; Van Steenberghe, D. Fixture design and overload influence marginal bone loss and future success in the Brånemark®system. *Clin. Oral. Implants Res.* **1992**, *3*, 104–111. [CrossRef] [PubMed]
16. Manor, Y.; Oubaid, S.; Mardinger, O.; Chaushu, G.; Nissan, J. Characteristics of Early Versus Late Implant Failure: A Retrospective Study. *J. Oral Maxillofac. Surg.* **2009**, *67*, 2649–2652. [CrossRef] [PubMed]
17. He, J.; Zhao, B.; Deng, C.; Shang, D.; Zhang, C. Assessment of Implant Cumulative Survival Rates in Sites with Different Bone Density and Related Prognostic Factors: An 8-Year Retrospective Study of 2,684 Implants. *Int. J. Oral Maxillofac. Implants* **2015**, *30*, 360–371. [CrossRef]
18. Vidyasagar, L.; Apse, P. Biological response to dental implant loading/overloading. Implant overloading: Empiricism or science. *Stomatologija* **2003**, *5*, 83–89.
19. Kim, Y.; Oh, T.J.; Misch, C.E.; Wang, H.L. Occlusal considerations in implant therapy: Clinical guidelines with biomechanical rationale. *Clin. Oral Implants Res.* **2005**, *16*, 26–35. [CrossRef]
20. Duyck, J.; Vandamme, K. The effect of loading on peri-implant bone: A critical review of the literature. *J. Oral Rehabil.* **2014**, *41*, 783–794. [CrossRef]
21. Koyano, K.; Esaki, D. Occlusion on oral implants: Current clinical guidelines. *J. Oral Rehabil.* **2015**, *42*, 153–161. [CrossRef] [PubMed]
22. Ayuso-Montero, R.; Mariano-Hernandez, Y.; Khoury-Ribas, L.; Rovira-Lastra, B.; Willaert, E.; Martinez-Gomis, J. Reliability and Validity of T-scan and 3D Intraoral Scanning for Measuring the Occlusal Contact Area. *J. Prosthodont.* **2020**, *29*, 19–25. [CrossRef]
23. Shopova, D.; Bozhkova, T.; Yordanova, S.; Yordanova, M. Case Report: Digital analysis of occlusion with T-Scan Novus in occlusal splint treatment for a patient with bruxism. *F1000Research* **2021**, *10*, 915. [CrossRef] [PubMed]
24. Gümüş, H.Ö.; Kılınç, H.İ.; Tuna, S.H.; Ozcan, N. Computerized analysis of occlusal contacts in bruxism patients treated with occlusal splint therapy. *J. Adv. Prosthodont.* **2013**, *5*, 256–261. [CrossRef] [PubMed]
25. Miyata, T.; Kobayashi, Y.; Araki, H.; Ohto, T.; Shin, K. The influence of controlled occlusal overload on peri-implant tissue. Part 3: A histologic study in monkeys. *Int. J. Oral Maxillofac. Implant.* **2000**, *15*, 425–431.
26. Isidor, F. Loss of osseointegration caused by occlusal load of oral implants: A clinical and radiographic study in monkeys. *Clin. Oral Implants Res.* **1996**, *7*, 143–152. [CrossRef] [PubMed]
27. Duyck, J.; Naert, I.; Rønold, H.J.; Ellingsen, J.E.; Van Oosterwyck, H.; Vander Sloten, J. The influence of static and dynamic loading on marginal bone reactions around osseointegrated implants: An animal experimental study. *Clin. Oral Implants Res.* **2001**, *12*, 207–218. [CrossRef]
28. Hürzeler, M.B.; Quiñones, C.R.; Kohal, R.J.; Rohde, M.; Strub, J.R.; Teuscher, U.; Caffesse, R.G. Changes in Peri-Implant Tissues Subjected to Orthodontic Forces and Ligature Breakdown in Monkeys. *J. Periodontol.* **1998**, *69*, 396–404. [CrossRef]
29. Heitz-Mayfield, L.J.; Schmid, B.; Weigel, C.; Gerber, S.; Bosshardt, D.D.; Jönsson, J.; Lang, N.P.; Jönsson, J. Does excessive occlusal load affect osseointegration? An experimental study in the dog. *Clin. Oral Implants Res.* **2004**, *15*, 259–268. [CrossRef]
30. Gotfredsen, K.; Berglundh, T.; Lindhe, J. Bone reactions adjacent to titanium implants subjected to static load: A study in the dog (I). *Clin. Oral Implants Res.* **2001**, *12*, 1–8. [CrossRef]
31. Page, M.J.; McKenzie, J.E.; Bossuyt, P.M.; Boutron, I.; Hoffmann, T.C.; Mulrow, C.D.; Shamseer, L.; Tetzlaff, J.M.; Akl, E.A.; Brennan, S.E.; et al. The PRISMA 2020 statement: An updated guideline for reporting systematic reviews. *BMJ* **2021**, *372*, 89.
32. Sterne, J.A.; Hernán, M.A.; Reeves, B.C.; Savovic, J.; Berkman, N.D.; Viswanathan, M.; Henry, D.; Altman, D.G.; Ansari, M.T.; Boutron, I.; et al. ROBINS-I: A tool for assessing risk of bias in non-randomised studies of interventions. *BMJ* **2016**, *355*, 4–10. [CrossRef]
33. Podaropoulos, L.; Veis, A.A.; Trisi, P.; Papadimitriou, S.; Alexandridis, C.; Kalyvas, D. Bone reactions around dental implants subjected to progressive static load: An experimental study in dogs. *Clin. Oral Implants Res.* **2016**, *27*, 910–917. [CrossRef] [PubMed]
34. Ferrari, D.S.; Piattelli, A.; Iezzi, G.; Faveri, M.; Rodrigues, J.A.; Shibli, J.A. Effect of lateral static load on immediately restored implants: Histologic and radiographic evaluation in dogs. *Clin. Oral Implants Res.* **2015**, *26*, e51–e56. [CrossRef] [PubMed]
35. Nagasawa, M.; Takano, R.; Maeda, T.; Uoshima, K. Observation of the Bone Surrounding an Overloaded Implant in a Novel Rat Model. *Int. J. Oral Maxillofac. Implants* **2013**, *28*, 109–116. [CrossRef]
36. Miyamoto, Y.; Koretake, K.; Hirata, M.; Kubo, T.; Akagawa, Y. Influence of static overload on the bony interface around implants in dogs. *Int. J. Prosthodont.* **2008**, *21*, 437–444.
37. Kozlovsky, A.; Tal, H.; Laufer, B.Z.; Leshem, R.; Rohrer, M.D.; Weinreb, M.; Artzi, Z. Impact of implant overloading on the peri-implant bone in inflamed and non-inflamed peri-implant mucosa. *Clin. Oral Implants Res.* **2007**, *18*, 601–610. [CrossRef]
38. Miyata, T.; Kobayashi, Y.; Araki, H.; Ohto, T.; Shin, K. The influence of controlled occlusal overload on peri-implant tissue. part 4: A histologic study in monkeys. *Int. J. Oral Maxillofac. Implants* **2002**, *17*, 384–390.
39. Asikainen, P.; Klemettil, E.; Vuilleminz, T.; Sutter, F.; Rainio, V.; Kotilainen, R. Titanium implants and lateral forces. *Clin. Oral Implants Res.* **1997**, *8*, 465–468. [CrossRef]

40. Isidor, F. Histological evaluation of peri-implant bone at implants subjected to occlusal overload or plaque accumulation. *Clin. Oral Implants Res.* **1997**, *8*, 1–9. [CrossRef]
41. Hoshaw, S.J.; Brunski, J.B.; Cochran, G.V.B. Mechanical loading of brånemark implants affects interfacial bone modeling and remodeling. *Int. J. Oral Maxillofac. Implants* **1994**, *9*, 1–33.
42. Ogiso, M.; Tabata, T.; Kuo, P.T.; Borghese, D. A histologic an occluded Prosthetics and Dental Implants comparison of the functional loading capacity of dense apatite implant and the natural dentition. *J. Prosthet. Dent.* **1994**, *71*, 581–588. [CrossRef]
43. Podaropoulos, L.; Trisi, P.; Papadimitriou, S.; Lazzara, R.; Kalyvas, D. The Influence of Progressive Study in Dogs. *Int. J. Oral Maxillofac. Implants* **2020**, *35*, 25–38. [CrossRef] [PubMed]
44. Lima, L.A.; Bosshardt, D.D.; Chambrone, L.; Araújo, M.G.; Lang, N.P. Excessive occlusal load on chemically modified and moderately rough titanium implants restored with cantilever reconstructions. An experimental study in dogs. *Clin. Oral Implant. Res.* **2019**, *30*, 1142–1154. [CrossRef]
45. Piccinini, M.; Cugnoni, J.; Botsis, J.; Ammann, P.; Wiskott, A. Peri-implant bone adaptations to overloading in rat tibiae: Experimental investigations and numerical predictions. *Clin. Oral Implant. Res.* **2016**, *27*, 1444–1453. [CrossRef]
46. Yagihara, A.; Kawasaki, R.; Mita, A.; Takakuda, K. Impact of Dynamic and Static Load on Bone Around Implants: An Experimental Study in a Rat Model. *Int. J. Oral Maxillofac. Implant.* **2016**, *31*, e49–e56. [CrossRef]
47. Maminskas, J.; Puisys, A.; Kuoppala, R.; Raustia, A.; Juodzbalys, G. The Prosthetic Influence and Biomechanics on Peri-Implant Strain: A Systematic Literature Review of Finite Element Studies. *J. Oral Maxillofac. Res.* **2016**, *7*, e4. [CrossRef]
48. Afrashtehfar, K.I.; Afrashtehfar, C.D. Lack of association between overload and peri-implant tissue loss in healthy conditions. *Evid. Based Dent.* **2016**, *17*, 92–93. [CrossRef]
49. Pellegrini, G.; Canullo, L.; Dellavia, C. Histological features of peri-implant bone subjected to overload. *Ann. Anat.-Anat. Anz.* **2016**, *206*, 57–63. [CrossRef]
50. Chang, M.; Chronopoulos, V.; Mattheos, N. Impact of excessive occlusal load on successfully-osseointegrated dental implants: A literature review. *J. Investig. Clin. Dent.* **2013**, *4*, 142–150. [CrossRef]
51. Rungruanganunt, P.; Taylor, T.D.; Eckert, S.E.; Karl, M. The effect of static load on dental implant survival: A systematic review. *Int. J. Oral Maxillofac. Implants* **2013**, *28*, 1218–1225. [CrossRef] [PubMed]
52. Naert, I.; Duyck, J.; Vandamme, K. Occlusal overload and bone/implant loss. *Clin. Oral Implants Res.* **2012**, *23* (Suppl. S6), 95–107. [CrossRef] [PubMed]
53. Sakka, S.; Baroudi, K.; Nassani, M.Z. Factors associated with early and late failure of dental implants. *J. Investig. Clin. Dent.* **2012**, *3*, 258–261. [CrossRef] [PubMed]
54. Hsu, Y.-T.; Fu, J.-H.; Al-Hezaimi, K.; Wang, H.-L. Biomechanical implant treatment complications: A systematic review of clinical studies of implants with at least 1 year of functional loading. *Int. J. Oral Maxillofac. Implants* **2012**, *27*, 894–904.
55. Chambrone, L.; Chambrone, L.A.; Lima, L.A. Effects of Occlusal Overload on Peri-Implant Tissue Health: A Systematic Review of Animal-Model Studies. *J. Periodontol.* **2010**, *81*, 1367–1378. [CrossRef]
56. Dănilă, V.; Augustin, M. Occlusal overload–a risk factor in implant based prostheses. *Rev. Med. Chir. Soc. Med. Nat. Iasi.* **2010**, *114*, 214–217.
57. Rilo, B.; da Silva, J.L.; Mora, M.J.; Santana, U. Guidelines for occlusion strategy in implant-borne prostheses. A review. *Int. Dent. J.* **2008**, *58*, 139–145. [CrossRef]
58. Hui, F.J.; Yap, A.U.J. Occlusion and periodontal disease—Where is the link? *Singapore Dent. J.* **2007**, *29*, 22–23.
59. Lobbezoo, F.; Brouwers, J.; Cune, M.; Naeije, M. Dental implants in patients with bruxing habits. *J. Oral Rehabil.* **2006**, *33*, 152–159. [CrossRef]
60. Isidor, F. Influence of forces on peri-implant bone. *Clin. Oral Implants Res.* **2006**, *17* (Suppl. S2), 8–18. [CrossRef]
61. Saadoun, A.P.; Le Gall, M.; Kricheck, M. Microbial infections and occlusal overload: Causes of failure in osseointegrated implants. *Pract. Periodontics Aesthet. Dent.* **1993**, *5*, 11–20.
62. Zandim-Barcelos, D.L.; Carvalho, G.G.; De Sapata, V.M.; Villar, C.C.; Hämmerle, C.; Romito, G.A. Implant-based factor as possible risk for peri-implantitis. *Braz. Oral Res.* **2019**, *33* (Suppl. S1), e067. [CrossRef] [PubMed]
63. Sadowsky, S.J. Occlusal overload with dental implants: A review. *Int. J. Implant Dent.* **2019**, *5*, 29. [CrossRef] [PubMed]
64. Naveau, A.; Shinmyouzu, K.; Moore, C.; Avivi-Arber, L.; Jokerst, J.; Koka, S. Etiology and Measurement of Peri-Implant Crestal Bone Loss (CBL). *J. Clin. Med.* **2019**, *8*, 166. [CrossRef] [PubMed]
65. Nuțu, E. Role of initial density distribution in simulations of bone remodeling around dental implants. *Acta Bioeng. Biomech.* **2018**, *20*, 23–31.
66. Eazhil, R.; Swaminathan, S.V.; Gunaseelan, M.; Kannan, G.V.; Alagesan, C. Impact of implant diameter and length on stress distribution in osseointegrated implants: A 3D FEA study. *J. Int. Soc. Prev. Community Dent.* **2016**, *6*, 590–596. [CrossRef]
67. Baggi, L.; Pastore, S.; Di Girolamo, M.; Vairo, G. Implant-bone load transfer mechanisms in complete-arch prostheses supported by four implants: A three-dimensional finite element approach. *J. Prosthet. Dent.* **2013**, *109*, 9–21. [CrossRef]
68. Baggi, L.; Cappelloni, I.; Di Girolamo, M.; Maceri, F.; Vairo, G. The influence of implant diameter and length on stress distribution of osseointegrated implants related to crestal bone geometry: A three-dimensional finite element analysis. *J. Prosthet. Dent.* **2008**, *100*, 422–431. [CrossRef]
69. Kitamura, E.; Stegaroiu, R.; Nomura, S.; Miyakawa, O. Influence of marginal bone resorption on stress around an implant—A three-dimensional finite element analysis. *J. Oral Rehabil.* **2005**, *32*, 279–286. [CrossRef]

70. Crupi, V.; Guglielmino, E.; La Rosa, G.; Vander Sloten, J.; Van Oosterwyck, H. Numerical analysis of bone adaptation around an oral implant due to overload stress. *Proc. Inst. Mech. Eng. Part H J. Eng. Med.* **2004**, *218*, 407–415. [CrossRef]
71. Watanabe, F.; Hata, Y.; Komatsu, S.; Ramos, T.C.; Fukuda, H. Finite element analysis of the influence of implant inclination, loading position, and load direction on stress distribution. *Odontology* **2003**, *91*, 31–36. [CrossRef] [PubMed]
72. Akça, K.; Iplikçioğlu, H. Finite element stress analysis of the influence of staggered versus straight placement of dental implants. *Int. J. Oral Maxillofac. Implants* **2001**, *16*, 722–730. [PubMed]
73. O'Mahony, A.; Bowles, Q.; Woolsey, G.; Robinson, S.J.; Spencer, P. Stress distribution in the single-unit osseointegrated dental implant: Finite element analyses of axial and off-axial loading. *Implant Dent.* **2000**, *9*, 207–218. [CrossRef] [PubMed]
74. Papavasiliou, G.; Kamposiora, P.; Bayne, S.C.; Felton, D.A. Three-dimensional finite elemente analysis of stress-distribution around single tooth implants as a function of bony support, prosthesis type, and loading durinf function. *J. Prosthet. Dent.* **1996**, *76*, 633–640. [CrossRef]
75. Chang, C.-L.; Chen, C.-S.; Yeung, T.C.; Hsu, M.-L. Biomechanical effect of a zirconia dental implant-crown system: A three-dimensional finite element analysis. *Int. J. Oral Maxillofac. Implant* **2012**, *27*, e49–e57.
76. Sridhar, S.; Wang, F.; Wilson, T.G.G.; Palmer, K.; Valderrama, P.; Rodrigues, D.C. The role of bacterial biofilm and mechanical forces in modulating dental implant failures. *J. Mech. Behav. Biomed. Mater.* **2019**, *92*, 118–127. [CrossRef]
77. Kan, J.P.M.; Judge, R.B.; Palamara, J.E.A. In vitro bone strain analysis of implant following occlusal overload. *Clin. Oral Implants Res.* **2014**, *25*, e73–e82. [CrossRef]
78. Nakashima, T.; Hayashi, M.; Fukunaga, T.; Kurata, K.; Oh-Hora, M.; Feng, J.Q.; Bonewald, L.F.; Kodama, T.; Wutz, A.; Wagner, E.F.; et al. Evidence for osteocyte regulation of bone homeostasis through RANKL expression. *Nat. Med.* **2011**, *17*, 1231–1234. [CrossRef]
79. Sheridan, R.A.; Decker, A.M.; Plonka, A.B.; Wang, H.-L. The Role of Occlusion in Implant Therapy: A Comprehensive Updated Review. *Implant Dent.* **2016**, *25*, 829–838. [CrossRef]
80. Hosokawa, R. Significance of occlusion for dental implant treatment. Clinical evidence of occlusion as a risk factor. *Nihon Hotetsu Shika Gakkai Zasshi* **2008**, *52*, 25–30. [CrossRef]
81. Passanezi, E.; Sant'Ana, A.C.P.; Damante, C.A. Occlusal trauma and mucositis or peri-implantitis? *J. Am. Dent. Assoc.* **2017**, *148*, 106–112. [CrossRef] [PubMed]
82. Mattheos, N.; Janda, M.S.; Zampelis, A.; Chronopoulos, V. Reversible, Non-plaque-induced loss of osseointegration of successfully loaded dental implants. *Clin. Oral Implants Res.* **2013**, *24*, 347–354. [CrossRef] [PubMed]
83. Tawil, G. Peri-implant bone loss caused by occlusal overload: Repair of the peri-implant defect following correction of the traumatic occlusion. A case report. *Int. J. Oral Maxillofac. Implant.* **2008**, *23*, 153–157.
84. Uribe, R.; Peñarrocha, M.; Sanchis, J.M.; García, O. Periimplantitis marginal por sobrecarga oclusal. A propósito de un caso Marginal peri-implantitis due to occlusal overload. A case. *Med. Oral Organo Of. Soc. Esp. Med. Oral. Acad. Iberoam. Patol. Med. Bucal* **2004**, *9*, 159–162.
85. Leung, K.C.M.; Chow, T.W.; Wat, P.Y.P.; Comfort, M.B. Peri-implant Bone Loss: Management of a Patient. *Int. J. Oral Maxillofac. Implant* **2001**, *16*, 273–277.
86. Rosenberg, E.S.; Torosian, J.P.; Slots, J. Microbial differences in 2 clinically distinct types of failures of osseointegrated implants. *Clin. Oral Implants Res.* **1991**, *2*, 135–144. [CrossRef]
87. Jofré, J.; Hamada, T.; Nishimura, M.; Klattenhoff, C. The effect of maximum bite force on marginal bone loss of mini-implants supporting a mandibular overdenture: A randomized controlled trial. *Clin. Oral Implants Res.* **2010**, *21*, 243–249. [CrossRef] [PubMed]
88. Naert, I.; Quirynen, M.; van Steenberghe, D.; Darius, P. A study of 589 consecutive implants supporting complete fixed prostheses. Part II: Prosthetic aspects. *J. Prosthet. Dent.* **1992**, *68*, 949–956. [CrossRef]
89. Chitumalla, R.; Kumari, K.H.; Mohapatra, A.; Parihar, A.S.; Anand, K.S.; Katragadda, P. Assessment of survival rate of dental implants in patients with bruxism: A 5-year retrospective study. *Contemp. Clin. Dent.* **2018**, *9*, S278–S282. [CrossRef]
90. Han, H.-J.; Kim, S.; Han, D.-H. Multifactorial Evaluation of Implant Failure: A 19-year Retrospective Study. *Int. J. Oral Maxillofac. Implants* **2014**, *29*, 303–310. [CrossRef]
91. Becker, C.M. Cantilever fixed prostheses utilizing dental implants: A 10-year retrospective analysis. *Quintessence Int.* **2004**, *35*, 437–441. [PubMed]
92. Lindquist, L.W.; Rockler, B.; Carlsson, G.E. Bone resorption around fixtures in edentulous patients treated with mandibular fixed tissue-integrated prostheses. *J. Prosthet. Dent.* **1988**, *59*, 59–63. [CrossRef]
93. Lindquist, L.W.; Carlsson, G.E.; Jemt, T. A prospective 15-year follow-up study of mandibular fixed prostheses supported by osseointegrated implants: Clinical results and marginal bone loss. *Clin. Oral Implants Res.* **1996**, *7*, 329–336. [CrossRef] [PubMed]
94. Carlsson, G.E.; Lindquist, L.W.; Jemt, T. Long-term marginal periimplant bone loss in edentulous patients. *Int. J. Prosthodont.* **2000**, *13*, 295–302. [PubMed]
95. Engel, E.; Gomez-Roman, G.; Axmann-Krcmar, D. Effect of occlusal wear on bone loss and Periotest value of dental implants. *Int. J. Prosthodont.* **2001**, *14*, 444–450.
96. Dalago, H.R.; Schuldt Filho, G.; Rodrigues, M.A.P.; Renvert, S.; Bianchini, M.A. Risk indicators for Peri-implantitis. A cross-sectional study with 916 implants. *Clin. Oral Implant. Res.* **2017**, *28*, 144–150. [CrossRef]

97. Kissa, J.; El Kholti, W.; Chemlali, S.; Kawtari, H.; Laalou, Y.; Albandar, J.M. Prevalence and risk indicators of peri-implant diseases in a group of Moroccan patients. *J. Periodontol.* **2021**, *92*, 1096–1106. [CrossRef]
98. Canullo, L.; Tallarico, M.; Radovanovic, S.; Delibasic, B.; Covani, U.; Rakic, M. Distinguishing predictive profiles for patient-based risk assessment and diagnostics of plaque induced, surgically and prosthetically triggered peri-implantitis. *Clin. Oral Implants Res.* **2016**, *27*, 1243–1250. [CrossRef]
99. Sadowsky, S.J. Mandibular implant-retained overdentures: A literature review. *J. Prosthet. Dent.* **2001**, *86*, 468–473. [CrossRef]
100. Sadowsky, S.J. Treatment considerations for maxillary implant overdentures: A systematic review. *J. Prosthet. Dent.* **2007**, *97*, 340–348. [CrossRef]
101. Klemetti, E. Is there a certain number of implants needed to retain an overdenture? *J. Oral Rehabil.* **2008**, *35*, 80–84. [CrossRef] [PubMed]
102. Nicolae, V.; Chiscop, I.; Cioranu, V.S.I.; Martu, M.A.; Luchian, A.I.; Martu, S.; Solomon, S.M. The use of photoactivated blue-o toluidine for periimplantitis treatment in patients with periodontal disease. *Rev. Chim. (Buchar.)* **2015**, *66*, 2121–2123.
103. Kerstein, R.B.; Radke, J. Clinician accuracy when subjectively interpreting articulating paper markings. *Cranio* **2014**, *32*, 13–23. [CrossRef] [PubMed]
104. Cenkoglu, B.G.; Balcioglu, N.B.; Ozdemir, T.; Mijiritsky, E. The Effect of the Length and Distribution of Implants for Fixed Prosthetic Reconstructions in the Atrophic Posterior Maxilla: A Finite Element Analysis. *Materials* **2019**, *12*, 2556. [CrossRef]
105. Farronato, D.; Manfredini, M.; Stevanello, A.; Campana, V.; Azzi, L.; Farronato, M. A Comparative 3D Finite Element Computational Study of Three Connections. *Materials* **2019**, *12*, 3135. [CrossRef]
106. Brune, A.; Stiesch, M.; Eisenburger, M.; Greuling, A. The effect of different occlusal contact situations on peri-implant bone stress—A contact finite element analysis of indirect axial loading. *Mater. Sci. Eng.* **2019**, *99*, 367–373. [CrossRef]

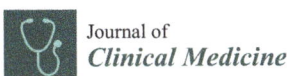

Journal of Clinical Medicine

Review

Effect of Toothpaste on the Surface Roughness of the Resin-Contained CAD/CAM Dental Materials: A Systematic Review

Adolfo Di Fiore [1,*], Edoardo Stellini [1], Michele Basilicata [2], Patrizio Bollero [2] and Carlo Monaco [3]

1. Department of Neuroscience, Section of Prosthetic and Digital Dentistry, University of Padova, 35122 Padova, Italy; edoardo.stellini@unipd.it
2. Department of Systems Medicine, University of Rome Tor Vergata, 00133 Roma, Italy; michele.basilicata@ptvonline.it (M.B.); patrizio.bollero@ptvonline.it (P.B.)
3. Department of Surgery, Medicine, and Dentistry, University of Modena e Reggio Emilia, 41121 Modena, Italy; carlo.monaco@unimore.it
* Correspondence: adolfo.difiore@unipd.it

Citation: Di Fiore, A.; Stellini, E.; Basilicata, M.; Bollero, P.; Monaco, C. Effect of Toothpaste on the Surface Roughness of the Resin-Contained CAD/CAM Dental Materials: A Systematic Review. *J. Clin. Med.* **2022**, *11*, 767. https://doi.org/10.3390/jcm11030767

Academic Editor: James Kit-hon Tsoi

Received: 19 January 2022
Accepted: 29 January 2022
Published: 31 January 2022

Publisher's Note: MDPI stays neutral with regard to jurisdictional claims in published maps and institutional affiliations.

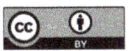

Copyright: © 2022 by the authors. Licensee MDPI, Basel, Switzerland. This article is an open access article distributed under the terms and conditions of the Creative Commons Attribution (CC BY) license (https:// creativecommons.org/licenses/by/ 4.0/).

Abstract: Background: The purpose of this review is to describe the possible effect of toothbrushing on surface roughness of resin-contained CAD/CAM materials. Methods: Systematic literature search for articles published in peer-reviewed journals between January 2000 and February 2020 has been conducted, which evaluated the effect of brushing on surface roughness of resin-contained CAD/CAM dental materials. The research was conducted in Scopus, PubMed/Medline, Web of Science, Embase, and Science Direct using a combination of the following MeSH/Emtree terms: "brushing", "resin-based", "dental", "CAD/CAM", and "surface roughness". Results: A total of 249 articles were found in the search during initial screening. Fifty-five articles were selected for the full-text evaluation after the steps of reading of abstract/title and remotion of duplicate. Only six articles fulfilled the inclusion criteria. The Cohen's Kappa agreement test showed an index of 0.91 for full-text. Discussion: Four of five selected articles identified an increase of surface roughness on resin-contained CAD/CAM materials after toothbrushing. Although all the articles examined used different toothpastes with no homogeneous relative dentine abrasivity (RDA) and cycles of brushing, the findings are about the same. The possible reason is attributable to the compositions of the resin-contained CAD/CAM materials. Conclusions: The surface roughness of most resin-contained CAD/CAM materials was affected by artificial toothbrushing. Correct knowledge of the composition of the dental material and toothpastes is fundamental to avoid an increase of surface roughness on prosthetic rehabilitation.

Keywords: CAD/CAM materials; toothbrushing wear; surface; roughness; surface integrity

1. Introduction

With growing awareness of esthetic rehabilitation, many patients require metal-free solutions [1]. Ceramic is the most used material for esthetic restorations in fixed prosthodontics. Surface roughness, translucency, resistance to wear, and mechanical properties are the main investigated characteristics of the ceramic surface [2]. In the last few years, computer-aided design/computer-aided manufacturing (CAD/CAM) has been introduced in the dentistry world and has improved the accuracy of prostheses, comfort for patients, and operative time [3,4]. Consequently, new different materials have been realized with different surfaces and mechanical behaviors [5,6]. The surface roughness is one of the factors that influenced the clinical survival of prosthetic rehabilitation, optical properties, wear of the antagonist teeth, and initiation of cracks [7]. Above the threshold Ra value of 0.2 μm for roughness, an increase of plaque accumulations has been observed on prosthetic materials [7]. The presence of bacteria on prosthetic rehabilitation becomes the main cause of biological complication, therefore, daily dental hygiene is necessary to remove plaque and prevent gingival inflammations [8]. Different factors influenced the surface roughness of the prosthetic materials, but the effect of brushing or polishing with toothpaste or prophylactic polishing pastes could be considered as one of the factors [9–11]. Regarding the polishing procedure by using the prophylactic pastes, several authors demonstrated the possible surface roughness alteration on prosthetic materials [10,11]. Few investigations on brushing are published [9]. However, most studies presented in the literature reported the abrasive effect of toothpaste and/or prophylactic pastes on the surface of composite materials and poly(methyl)methacrylate resin materials [12–16]. Commercially, resin-based CAD/CAM materials are used to produce prosthetic rehabilitation, moreover, different kinds of toothpastes are available with different relative dentine abrasivity (RDA indexes) [17]. However, few studies investigated the effect of brushing on these new materials. So, the purpose of this systematic review was to assess the effect of toothpaste on the surface roughness of the resin-contained CAD/CAM dental materials.

2. Materials and Methods

This systematic review was conducted in accordance with the Preferred Reporting Items for Systematic Reviews statement [18]. The PICO question was: "In the resin-contained CAD/CAM dental material (P), does the use of toothpaste (I) have any possible adverse effects (C) in terms of surface roughness modifications (O)?".

2.1. Search Strategy

Electronic database searches of MEDLINE, EMBASE, Web of Science, Science Direct and Scopus were performed using the following keywords and MeSH/Emtree terms based on a search strategy used for searching MEDLINE: "brushing", "resin-based", "dental", "CAD/CAM", and "surface roughness". In addition, a manual search of the bibliographies of the most relevant systematic reviews and of all included and excluded articles was employed to identify other eligible studies.

2.2. Screening Method and Data Extraction

Titles and abstracts were screened, and the full texts of all potentially relevant publications were reviewed independently by the two authors (A.D.F., E.S.). Any disagreements between the two reviewers regarding inclusion were resolved by discussion. Cohen's Kappa statistic was calculated after the full-texts examination. The investigators recorded the study title, authors, year of publication, journal in which the research was published, study type (in vitro or in vivo research), brushing procedure (i.e., toothpaste, RDA, timing), prosthetic materials investigated, and surface roughness values before and after brushing.

2.3. Inclusion and Exclusion Criteria

The inclusion criteria were confined to full-text articles in English, published in peer-reviewed journals between 1 January 2000 and 28 February 2020, which evaluated the effect of brushing on surface roughness of resin-contained CAD/CAM dental materials. The exclusion criteria were articles that described other adverse effects than surface roughness, polishing procedure, letters to the editor, personal communications, reviews and meta-analyses. Surface roughness was the primary factor evaluated in each article. Subsequently, scientific articles that brought a better understanding of the different adverse effects of brushing on resin-contained CAD/CAM dental materials were identified to clarify and add knowledge.

2.4. Quality Assessment

The quality of each included study was individually evaluated following the Cochrane Collaboration guidelines. The Risk of Bias in Non-randomized Studies of Interventions (ROBINS-I) tool was utilized [19]. Each included study was classified as "low", "moderate", "serious" or "critical" risk of bias. Then, an overall score was given, judging the study at "low risk of bias" when it was assessed "low" in all domains, at "moderate risk of bias" when it was assessed "low" or "moderate" in all domains, at "serious risk of bias" when it was assessed "serious" in at least one domain or at "critical risk of bias" when it was assessed "critical" in at least one domain.

3. Results

A total of 249 articles were found in the search during the initial screening. Two hundred and nine records were identified through database searching and 40 from the manual search. After duplicate studies had been removed, 198 records were screened. After title/abstract evaluation, 55 articles were selected for the full-text evaluation, of which six fulfilled the inclusion criteria (Figure 1).

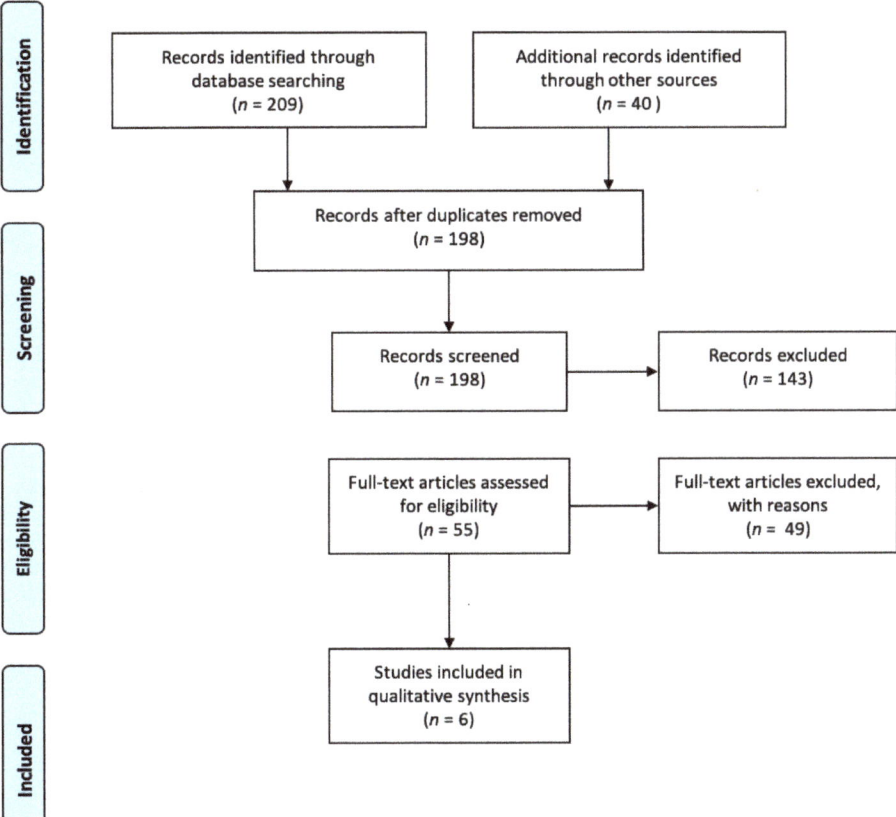

Figure 1. PRISMA flow chart of screened, withdrawn and included articles through the review process.

The main reasons for exclusion were that several studies investigated the effect of toothbrushing on direct composite and ceramic materials. The Cohen's Kappa agreement test showed an index of 0.91 for full-text for the articles selected. Six articles were selected according to the inclusion criteria [20–25]. No clinical studies were included. All six articles investigated Lava Ultimate (3M Espe) and Vita Enamic (Vita Zahnfabrik). Three included the Cerasmart (GC, GC Europe NV) [21,23,24], two Gradia Block (GC) and Shofu Block Hc (Shofu) [21,23], one on Katana Avencia (Kuraray Noritake) [21], Paradigm

MZ100 (3M ESPE) [22], Ambarino High Class (Creamed) [22], and Hybrid Resin Block (Yamamoto) [23]. All authors analyzed the surface roughness with a profilometer before and after the procedure of toothbrushing by using a toothbrush machine. Flury et al. [22] performed 3 measurements for specimen over a transverse length of Lt = 5.600 mm with a cut-off value of 0.8 mm and a stylus speed of 0.5 mm/second. Kamonkhantikul et al. [23] measured the sample tracing a length of 2 mm with a speed of 500 μm/s, and a cut-off length of 0.25. Five parallel measurements, each 400 μm apart, were performed perpendicular to the toothbrushing direction. Instead, Schmitt de Andrade et al. [24] made three profile measurements for each specimen for 4.2 mm along the specimen's surface with a cut-off value of 0.25 mm and a stylus speed of 0.1 mm/s. No details on measurements with the profilometer were reported in the article of Morman et al. [20] and Koizumi et al. [21]. Nima et al. [25] used a 3D noncontact laser-scanning microscope to obtain the measurements and 3D images of the sample. All authors used the mean surface roughness (Ra) value in μm to compare the value before and after toothbrushing [20–24] except Nima et al. [25], who used the maximum relative depth (Rv). For Rv calculation, five measurements were made that started in the control area and extended into the brushed region.

Different toothpastes were used in the experiments. RDA index values were 70 for the toothpaste used by Flury et al. [22], 136 in the research of Koizumi et al. [21], 80 for Kamonkhantikul et al. [23], 70/80 for Schmitt de Andrade et al. [24], 44 for Nima et al. [25], and not identified in the article of Morman et al. [20]. Five of six selected articles identified an increase of surface roughness on resin-contained CAD/CAM materials after toothbrushing [21–25]. Some materials such as Cerasmart (GC) [21–23] and Shofu Block Hc (Shofu) [21,23] were more affected by toothbrushing than others such as Lava Ultimate (3M Espe) and Vita Enamic (Vita Zahnfabrik). Regarding the cycles of artificial toothbrushing, several frequencies were performed. Flury et al. [22] applied 3000 cycles that are equivalent to 6000 toothbrushing strokes. Koizumi et al. [21] applied the specimen to 20,000 reciprocal strokes (approximately 120 min), 40,000 cycles were applied by Kamonkhantiku et al. [23], and 1500 cycles for Morman et al. [20]. Instead, Schmitt de Andrade et al. [24] carried out 100,000 toothbrushing strokes and Nima et al. [25] submitted the sample to 300,000 toothbrushing strokes (150 cycles/min).

All data regarding authors, type of studies, toothbrushing test, and surface roughness analysis are reported in Table 1.

The risk of bias in six studies included was classified as moderate risk of bias (Table 2). Three studies [22–25] were deemed to have "low risk of bias" for selection of the major resin-contained CAD/CAM materials present in the dental market and for detailed description of the methods and results. The other three studies [20,21] were considered as "moderate risk of bias" due to the use of ceramic materials during the investigation and some missing data in the methodology used during the experimentations.

Table 1. Data collection.

Authors	Year	Study Design	Sample	Toothbrushing Test	Surface Roughness Analysis	Roughness Parameter Measured	Correlation Toothbrushing and Surface Roughness
Morman et al. [20]	2013	In vitro	Lava Ultimate (3M ESPE) Vita Enamic (Vita Zahnfabrik)	Toothbrush Machine unspecified	Profilometer (Form Talysurf S2, Taylor Hobson, England).	Ra (µm)	NO
Koizumi et al. [21]	2015	In vitro	Vita Enamic (Vita Zahnfabrik) Gradia Block (GC) Shofu Block Hc (Shofu) Lava Ultimate (3M ESPE) Katana Avencia (Kuraray Noritake) Cerasmart (GC)	Toothbrush machine (K236, Tokyo Giken)	Profilometer (Surfcom 1400A, Tokyo Seimitsu, Tokyo, Japan)	Ra (µm) Rz (µm)	YES (Cerasmart and Shofu Block) NO (other materials)
Flury et al. [22]	2016	In vitro	Paradigm MZ100 (3M ESPE) Lava Ultimate (3M ESPE) Vita Enamic (Vita Zahnfabrik) Ambarino High Class (Creamed)	Toothbrush machine (Syndicad LR1)	Profilometer (Perthometer S2; Mahr GmbH)	Ra (µm) Rz (µm)	YES (Ambarino) NO (Lava Ultimate and Vita Enamic)
Kamonkhantikul et al. [23]	2016	In vitro	Shofu Block Hc (Shofu) Cerasmart (GC) Gradia Block (GC) Hybrid Resin Block (Yamamoto) Lava Ultimate (3M ESPE) Vita Enamic (Vita Zahnfabrik)	Toothbrush machine (V-8 Cross Brushing Machine, SABRI Dental)	Profilometer (Talyscan 150, Taylor Hobson, Leicester, England)	Ra (µm)	YES
Schmitt de Andrade et al. [24]	2021	In vitro	Cerasmart (GC) Vita Enamic (Vita Zahnfabrik) Lava Ultimate (3M ESPE)	Toothbrush machine (MEV2; Odeme Dental Research)	Contact profilometer (MaxSurf XT 20; Mahr).	Ra (µm)	YES
Nima et al. [25]	2021	In vitro	Vita Enamic (Vita Zahnfabrik) Lava Ultimate (3M ESPE)	Toothbrush machine (Maquina de Escivaca; Biopdi)	A 3D noncontact laser-scanning microscope (LEXT OLES4000 3D; Olympus).	Rv (µm)	YES

Table 2. Risk of bias assessment (ROBINS-I).

Study	Pre-Intervention		At Intervention		Post-Intervention			Overall Risk of Bias
	Confounding	Selection	Classification of Intervention	Deviation From intended Intervention	Missing Data	Measurement of Outcome	Reporting Result	
Morman et al. [20]	M	M	L	M	S	M	M	M
Koizumi et al. [21]	M	L	M	M	S	M	L	M
Flury et al. [22]	L	L	L	M	L	L	L	L
Kamonkhantikul et al. [23]	L	M	M	L	L	L	L	L
Schmitt de Andrade et al. [24]	L	M	L	M	L	L	L	L
Nima et al. [25]	L	M	M	L	L	L	L	L

L = "low risk of bias"; M = "moderate risk of bias"; S = "serious risk of bias"; C = "critical risk of bias".

4. Discussion

The systematic review reported the relationship between toothpaste, RDA index, and surface roughness (Ra) for five articles [20–24] and maximum relative depth (Rv) for one [25] on resin-contained CAD/CAM dental materials.

Flury et al. [22] investigated the effect of artificial toothbrushing on the CAD/CAM materials including different resin containing dental materials such as Lava Ultimate (3M ESPE), Vita Enamic (Vita Zahnfabrik), and Ambarino High-Class (Creamed). All the materials were stored in tap water in an incubator for 6 months at 37 °C. Each month all the samples were undergoing artificial toothbrushing for 500 cycles using a toothbrushing machine. The surfaces' roughness was measured by using a profilometer before and after the procedures of storage and toothbrushing. The findings demonstrated different behaviors of the resin-contained CAD/CAM materials. The surface roughness (Ra) significantly increased after artificial toothbrushing and storage for Ambarino High-Class (Ra and Rz, $p < 0.001$). Instead, Lava Ultimate and Vita Enamic showed no significant change in surface roughness after artificial toothbrushing and storage compared with after polishing ($p > 0.05$). The reason could be explained by the different filling materials used to compose the blocks. The Ambarino High-Class presents a 70 weight % ceramic-like inorganic silicate glass filler particles and 30 weight % highly cross-linked polymer blends, the Lava Ultimate has 80 weight % (65 vol%) nanoceramic particles (zirconia filler (4–11 nm), silica filler (20 nm), aggregated zirconia/silica cluster filler), 20 weight % (35 vol%) highly cross-linked (methacrylate-based) polymer matrix, and the Vita Enamic is composed of a 86 weight % feldspathic-based ceramic network and 14 weight % acrylate polymer network (infiltrated into feldspathic-based ceramic network). The first difference that emerged among the blocks is the low percentage of the matrix which is below 20% in the materials that did not change the surface roughness after toothbrushing.

Koizumi et al. [21] tested six different "resin-ceramic" CAD/CAM materials such as Vita Enamic (Vita Zahnfabrik), Gradia Block (GC), Shofu Block HC (Shofu), Lava Ultimate (3M ESPE), Katana Avencia block (Kuraray Noritake Dental), and Cerasmart (GC) after simulating a toothbrushing of five years. The profilometer was used to detect the surface roughness. The results showed a significant difference, regarding the Ra, in the Cerasmart and Shofu Block HC materials after toothbrush abrasion compared with the control group represented by the ceramic (Vita Marks II, Vita Zahnfabrik). Also, these findings are conducible to the "nanofillers" type, not only to the inorganic filler contents but also filler size, filler form, and polymeric matrix [26]. Kamonkhantikul et al. [23] tested the surface roughness of six resin-contained CAD/CAM materials such as Shofu Block Hc (Shofu), Cerasmart (GC), Gradia Block (GC), Hybrid Resin, Block (Yamamoto), Lava Ultimate (3M, ESPE), and Vita Enamic (Vita Zahnfabrik) after 40,000 cycles of toothbrushing. The statistical analyses indicated that significant differences were found in Ra between the measuring stages for each material tested except for the Gradia Block (GC) and Vita Enamic (Vita Zahnfabrik). The authors attributed the differences in wear to the chemical compositions. The Gradia Block (GC) consists of large irregularly shaped silicate glass and numerous pre-polymerized filler particles that could possibly protect its soft resin matrix from toothbrushing, instead the Vita Enamic (Vita Zahnfabrik) is constructed with ceramic filler. However, the conclusions reported that all materials present an acceptable toothbrush wear resistance.

No relationships between toothbrushing and surface roughness (Ra) emerged in the study conducted by Mormon et al. [20]. The investigated samples include Lava Ultimate (3M ESPE), Vita Enamic (Vita Zahnfabrik), and other ceramic blocks such as zirconia and lithium disilicate. All the specimens were stored for 7 days in 37 °C deionized water, and successively were mounted in a toothbrushing machine for 40,000 cycles. However, the authors concluded that the experimental toothbrushing wear in the present study significantly reduced the gloss of enamel and of all material specimens, except zirconium dioxide ceramic. Instead, de Andrade et al. [24] determined significant differences among the chairside CAD-CAM materials and simulated toothbrushing. The authors submitted the sample to 100,000 brushing strokes, which simulated 10 years of clinical wear. The sample analyzed was composed of IPS Empress CAD (Ivoclar Vivadent AG), Cerasmart (GC), Vita Enamic (Vita Zahnfabrik), Lava Ultimate (3M, ESPE), and Grandio Block (VOCO GmbH). After brushing, the IPS Empress CAD (Ivoclar Vivadent AG) showed the lowest Ra values, followed by the Lava Ultimate (3M, ESPE) and the Vita Enamic (Vita Zahnfabrik). Instead, the other materials have the highest Ra values after brushing. Indeed, the Cerasmart (GC) and Grandio Block (VOCO GmbH) reached mean roughness values higher than the threshold Ra value of 0.2 µm reported in the literature [27].

Nima et al. [25] submitted ten specimens of Vita Enamic (Vita Zahnfabrik) and Lava Ultimate (3M, ESPE) to 300,000 toothbrushing strokes. The results showed an increase in roughness (Rv = maximum relative depth) and gloss before and after toothbrushing. Although all the articles examined used different toothpastes with no homogeneous RDA, different toothbrushing machine, and cycles of brushing, the findings are about the same. Some authors tested the resin-contained CAD/CAM materials from 40,000 cycles to 1500 cycles [20–25]. Koizumi et al. [21] brushed the specimens for 120 min (20,000 cycles). Assuming that the ideal time for toothbrushing is 120 s two times a day [28,29], the 20,000 cycles may correspond to an amount of five years. However, in literature the articles reported that the actual mean brushing time is 65.2 to 83.5 s per day [29]. Therefore, the studies may correspond to a clinical simulation with a range of 1 to 20 years. Regarding the different granulometry present in the toothpastes, the authors used different RDA index values in the experiments, which influenced the surface roughness of the resin-contained CAD/CAM materials investigated in the articles in the same ways [18–23]. The reason for this comportment is attributable to the compositions of the resin-contained CAD/CAM materials. Indeed, blocks such as Lava Ultimate present 69% SiO_2 and 31% ZrO_2 fillers that improve the surface resistance to wear and the slight change in surface roughness after toothbrushing were considered clinically acceptable [21,22]. The aspect of the surface roughness remains a difficulty that clinicians do not consider. The literature reported 0.2 µm as the threshold value above which the plaque accumulation on dental materials increase [27]. However, it is difficult to measure the value clinically and no authors assessed the bristles' effects on the materials. Therefore, a correct knowledge of the composition of dental material and the possible effect of toothbrushing is fundamental to obtain success and survival of the prosthetic rehabilitations. In summary, the main limitation encountered in the majority of the included studies consists of the assessment of resin-contained CAD/CAM material only in vitro studies without including the different clinical aspects such as saliva, blood, different types of beverages, and the daily comportment of patients. Other drawbacks of this systematic review have been the lack of studies in this field, however, the results of the articles highlighted the effect of toothbrushing on resin-contained CAD/CAM materials. New clinical and in vitro studies are needed to improve the dental hygiene of our patients and to prevent the increase of pathologies that correlate to plaque accumulation.

5. Conclusions

With the limitations of this study, we can conclude that the surface roughness of most resin-contained CAD/CAM materials was affected by artificial toothbrushing. Therefore, a correct knowledge of the composition of the dental material and toothpastes is fundamental to avoid an increase of surface roughness on the prosthetic rehabilitations. Moreover, future clinical studies are needed to assess the behavior of resin-contained CAD/CAM materials in clinic situations.

Author Contributions: Conceptualization, A.D.F.; methodology, A.D.F.; validation, E.S., P.B. and C.M.; investigation, A.D.F. and E.S.; data curation, A.D.F.; writing—original draft preparation, A.D.F.; writing—review and editing, C.M. and M.B.; supervision, E.S. All authors have read and agreed to the published version of the manuscript.

Funding: This research received no external funding.

Institutional Review Board Statement: Not applicable.

Informed Consent Statement: Not applicable.

Data Availability Statement: Not applicable.

Conflicts of Interest: The authors declare no conflict of interest.

References

1. Reich, S.; Wichmann, M.; Nkenke, E.; Proeschel, P. Clinical fit of all-ceramic three-unit fixed partial dentures, generated with three different CAD/CAM systems. *Eur. J. Oral Sci.* **2005**, *113*, 174–179. [CrossRef] [PubMed]
2. Aykent, F.; Yondem, I.; Ozyesil, A.G.; Gunal, S.K.; Avunduk, M.C.; Ozkan, S. Effect of different finishing techniques for restorative materials on surface roughness and bacterial adhesion. *J. Prosthet. Dent.* **2010**, *103*, 221–227. [CrossRef]
3. Di Fiore, A.; Vigolo, P.; Graiff, L.; Stellini, E. Digital vs. Conventional Workflow for Screw-Retained Single-Implant Crowns: A Comparison of Key Considerations. *Int. J. Prosthodont.* **2018**, *31*, 577–579. [CrossRef]
4. Granata, S.; Giberti, L.; Vigolo, P.; Stellini, E.; Di Fiore, A. Incorporating a facial scanner into the digital workflow: A dental technique. *J. Prosthet. Dent.* **2020**, *123*, 781–785. [CrossRef] [PubMed]
5. Strasser, T.; Preis, V.; Behr, M.; Rosentritt, M. Roughness, surface energy, and superficial damages of CAD/CAM materials after surface treatment. *Clin. Oral Investig.* **2018**, *22*, 2787–2797. [CrossRef] [PubMed]
6. Arena, A.; Prete, F.; Rambaldi, E.; Bignozzi, M.C.; Monaco, C.; Di Fiore, A.; Chevalier, J. Nanostructured Zirconia-Based Ceramics and Composites in Dentistry: A State-of-the-Art Review. *Nanomaterials* **2019**, *9*, 1393. [CrossRef]
7. Checketts, M.R.; Turkyilmaz, I.; Asar, N.V. An investigation of the effect of scaling-induced surface roughness on bacterial adhesion in common fixed dental restorative materials. *J. Prosthet. Dent.* **2014**, *112*, 1265–1270. [CrossRef]
8. Bressan, E.; Tessarolo, F.; Sbricoli, L.; Caola, I.; Nollo, G.; Di Fiore, A. Effect of chlorhexidine in preventing plaque biofilm on healing abutment: A crossover controlled study. *Implant Dent.* **2014**, *23*, 64–68. [CrossRef]
9. Garza, L.A.; Thompson, G.; Cho, S.H.; Berzins, D.W. Effect of toothbrushing on shade and surface roughness of extrinsically stained pressable ceramics. *J. Prosthet. Dent.* **2016**, *115*, 489–494. [CrossRef]
10. Monaco, C.; Arena, A.; Özcan, M. Effect of prophylactic polishing pastes on roughness and translucency of lithium disilicate ceramic. *Int. J. Periodontics Restor. Dent.* **2014**, *34*, 26–29. [CrossRef]
11. Monaco, C.; Arena, A.; Scheda, L.; Di Fiore, A.; Zucchelli, G. In vitro 2D and 3D roughness and spectrophotometric and gloss analyses of ceramic materials after polishing with different prophylactic pastes. *J. Prosthet. Dent.* **2020**, *124*, 787.e1–787.e8. [CrossRef] [PubMed]
12. Neme, A.M.; Wagner, W.C.; Pink, F.E.; Frazier, K.B. The effect of prophylactic polishing pastes and toothbrushing on the surface roughness of resin composite materials in vitro. *Oper. Dent.* **2003**, *28*, 808–815. [PubMed]
13. Liljeborg, A.; Tellefsen, G.; Johannsen, G. The use of a profilometer for both quantitative and qualitative measurements of toothpaste abrasivity. *Int. J. Dent. Hyg.* **2010**, *8*, 237–243. [CrossRef] [PubMed]
14. Gungor, H.; Gundogdu, M.; Duymus, Z.Y. Investigation of the effect of different polishing techniques on the surface roughness of denture base and repair materials. *J. Prosthet. Dent.* **2014**, *112*, 1271–1277. [CrossRef] [PubMed]
15. Sahin, O.; Koroglu, A.; Dede, D.Ö.; Yilmaz, B. Effect of surface sealant agents on the surface roughness and color stability of denture base materials. *J. Prosthet. Dent.* **2016**, *116*, 610–616. [CrossRef]
16. Yurdaguven, H.; Aykor, A.; Ozel, E.; Sabuncu, H.; Soyman, M. Influence of a prophylaxis paste on surface roughness of different composites, porcelain, enamel and dentin surfaces. *Eur. J. Dent.* **2012**, *6*, 1–8. [CrossRef]
17. Hamza, B.; Attin, T.; Cucuzza, C.; Gubler, A.; Wegehaupt, F.J. RDA and REA Values of Commercially Available Toothpastes Utilising Diamond Powder and Traditional Abrasives. *Oral Health Prev. Dent.* **2020**, *18*, 807–814.
18. Moher, D.; Liberati, A.; Tetzlaff, J.; Altman, D.G.; PRISMA Group. Prefered reporting items for systematic reviews and meta-analyses: The PRISMA statement. *J. Clin. Epidemiol.* **2009**, *62*, 1006–1012. [CrossRef]
19. Sterne, J.A.; Hernán, M.A.; Reeves, B.C.; Savović, J; Berkman, N. D.; Viswanathan, M.; Henry, D.; Altman, D.G.; Ansari, M.T.; Boutron, I.; et al. ROBINS-I: A tool for assessing risk of bias in non-randomised studies of interventions. *BMJ* **2016**, *355*, i4919. [CrossRef]
20. Mörmann, W.H.; Stawarczyk, B.; Ender, A.; Sener, B.; Attin, T.; Mehl, A. Wear characteristics of current aesthetic dental restorative CAD/CAM materials: Two-body wear, gloss retention, roughness and Martens hardness. *J. Mech. Behav. Biomed. Mater.* **2013**, *20*, 113–125. [CrossRef]
21. Koizumi, H.; Saiki, O.; Nogawa, H.; Hiraba, H.; Okazaki, T.; Matsumura, H. Surface roughness and gloss of current CAD/CAM resin composites before and after toothbrush abrasion. *Dent. Mater. J.* **2015**, *34*, 881–887. [CrossRef] [PubMed]
22. Flury, S.; Diebold, E.; Peutzfeldt, A.; Lussi, A. Effect of artificial toothbrushing and water storage on the surface roughness and micromechanical properties of tooth-colored CAD-CAM materials. *J. Prosthet. Dent.* **2017**, *117*, 767–774. [CrossRef] [PubMed]
23. Kamonkhantikul, K.; Arksornnukit, M.; Lauvahutanon, S.; Takahashi, H. Toothbrushing alters the surface roughness and gloss of composite resin CAD/CAM blocks. *Dent. Mater. J.* **2016**, *35*, 225–232. [CrossRef] [PubMed]
24. de Andrade, G.S.; Augusto, M.G.; Simões, B.V.; Pagani, C.; Saavedra, G.S.F.A.; Bresciani, E. Impact of simulated toothbrushing on surface properties of chairside CAD-CAM materials: An in vitro study. *J. Prosthet. Dent.* **2021**, *125*, 469.e1–469.e6. [CrossRef]

25. Nima, G.; Lugo-Varillas, J.G.; Soto, J.; Faraoni, J.J.; Palma-Dibb, R.G.; Correa-Medina, A.; Giannini, M. Effect of toothbrushing on the surface of enamel, direct and indirect CAD/CAM restorative materials. *Int. J. Prosthodont.* **2021**, *34*, 473–481. [CrossRef]
26. Ferracane, J.L.; Mitchem, J.C.; Condon, J.R.; Todd, R. Wear and marginal breakdown of composites with various degrees of cure. *J. Dent. Res.* **1997**, *76*, 1508–1516. [CrossRef]
27. Bollen, C.M.; Lambrechts, P.; Quirynen, M. Comparison of surface roughness of oral hard materials to the threshold surface roughness for bacterial plaque retention: A review of the literature. *Dent. Mater.* **1997**, *13*, 258–269. [CrossRef]
28. Dentino, A.R.; Derderian, G.; Wolf, M.; Cugini, M.; Johnson, R.; Van Swol, R.L.; King, D.; Marks, P.; Warren, P. Six-month comparison of powered versus manual toothbrushing for safety and efficacy in the absence of professional instruction in mechanical plaque control. *J. Periodontol.* **2002**, *73*, 770–778. [CrossRef]
29. Creeth, J.E.; Gallagher, A.; Sowinski, J.; Bowman, J.; Barrett, K.; Lowe, S.; Patel, K.; Bosma, M.L. The effect of brushing time and dentifrice on dental plaque removal in vivo. *J. Dent. Hyg.* **2009**, *83*, 111–116.

Article

Association between Peri-Implant Soft Tissue Health and Different Prosthetic Emergence Angles in Esthetic Areas: Digital Evaluation after 3 Years' Function

Diego Lops [1], Eugenio Romeo [1], Stefano Calza [2], Antonino Palazzolo [1], Lorenzo Viviani [3], Stefano Salgarello [3], Barbara Buffoli [4,*] and Magda Mensi [3]

1. Department of Prosthodontics, Dental Clinic, School of Dentistry, University of Milan, 20100 Milan, Italy
2. Unit of Biostatistics and Bioinformatics, Department of Molecular and Translational Medicine, University of Brescia, 25121 Brescia, Italy
3. Department of Surgical Specialties, Dental Clinic, School of Dentistry, University of Brescia, 25125 Brescia, Italy
4. Section of Anatomy and Physiopathology, Department of Clinical and Experimental Sciences, University of Brescia, Viale Europa 11, 25123 Brescia, Italy
* Correspondence: barbara.buffoli@unibs.it; Tel.: +39-030-3717479

Abstract: Background: The aim of the present retrospective study was to assess peri-implant soft tissue health for implants restored with different prosthetic emergence profile angles. Methods: Patients were treated with implants supporting fixed dentures and were followed for 3 years. Buccal emergence angle (EA) measured at 3 years of follow-up visits (t1) were calculated for two different groups: Group 1 (153 implants) for restorations with angle between implant axis and prosthetic emergence angle from $\geq 30°$, and Group 2 (67 implants) for those with angle $\leq 30°$, respectively. Image J software was used for the measurements. Moreover, peri-implant soft tissue parameters such as pocket probing depth (PPD), plaque index (PI) and gingival index (GI) were assessed, respectively. Results: A total of 57 patients were included in the analysis and a total of 220 implants were examined. Mean ($\pm$SD) EA in Groups 1 and 2 was 46.4 ± 12.2 and 24.5 ± 4.7 degrees, respectively. After 3 years of follow-up, a PPD difference of 0.062 mm ($CI_{95\%}$ -0.041 mm; 0.164 mm) was calculated between the two groups and was not statistically significant ($p = 0.238$). Similar results were found for PI (OR = 0.78, $CI_{95\%}$ 0.31; 1.98, $p = 0.599$). Furthermore, GI scores of 2 and 3 were found for nine implants (5.9%) in Group 1, and for five implants in Group 2 (7.5%). A non-significant difference ($p = 0.76$) was found. Conclusions: Peri-implant soft-tissue health does not seem to be influenced by EA itself, when a proper emergence profile is provided for implant-supported reconstructions in anterior areas.

Keywords: dental implant; emergence angle; retrospective study; sub-crestal placement; emergence profile

1. Introduction

A critical role in dental implant aesthetic and functional long-term prognosis is played by peri-implant soft tissues. Mucosal level stability after implant placement could be affected by soft tissue quality and quantity, type of surgical procedure [1] and prosthetic design [2]. Peri-implant soft tissue is composed of well-keratinized oral epithelium, sulcular epithelium, and junctional epithelium, as well as underlying connective tissue. The role of an adequate band of keratinized mucosa around dental implants has been widely investigated in the literature. Even then, higher values of mucosa recession and loss of attachment were correlated with inadequate width of keratinized mucosa [3–5]. Keratinized oral epithelium continues in the sulcular epithelium and then in the junctional epithelium; this is a non-keratinized epithelium that, due to its unique structural and functional adaptation, plays a critical role in maintaining periodontal health by forming the front line of defense against periodontal bacterial infection. Moreover, peri-implant tissue architecture may be influenced by prosthetic emergence profile (EP) design [6,7]. Emergence profile was defined as the contour of a tooth or restoration, such as the crown on a natural tooth, dental implant, or dental implant abutment, as it relates to the emergence from circumscribed soft tissues [8]. Additionally, emergence profile zones were classified [9] in order to describe their importance in peri-implant tissue shaping and fulfilling aesthetic outcomes. Among such aesthetic criteria, interproximal papilla contour, gingival margin scalloping and buccal soft tissue thickness should be considered [10]. In addition, soft tissue architecture may contribute to preventing peri-implant soft tissue inflammation, giving patients real chances to follow proper oral hygiene indications [11]. Not only has a peri-implant tissue inflammation index addressed an adequate emergence profile, but also a proper emergence angle (EA) selection [12].

EA was reported as the angle between the average tangent of the transitional contour relative to the long axis of a tooth [8]. It was suggested by Katafuchi et al. [12] not to overcome a 30° EA value to preserve soft tissue health in the transition zone (Figure 1).

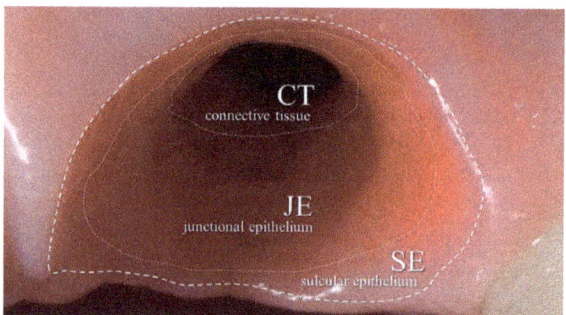

Figure 1. Peri-implant transition zone: connective tissue CT (1–1.5 mm) is directly connected to the peri-implant bone tissue. A junctional epithelium JE (1–2 mm) with a non-keratinized epithelium can be found above CT. A stratified squamous epithelium corresponding to the sulcular epithelium SE (1–1.5 mm) provides for the gingival margin area and is more superficial than both CT and JE, respectively.

On the other hand, in a 3-year follow-up report, no direct correlation between MBL (marginal bone level) change and emergence angles was found by Lops et al. [10]. Moreover, limited evidence about this correlation was highlighted by Mattheos et al. [13] in a critical review.

Due to the lack of agreement on this topic, more qualitative and quantitative data are needed to set further conclusions. Therefore, the primary outcome of the present report was to investigate any correlation between prosthetic emergence angles (<30° and ≥30°) and probing pocket depth (PPD) for implants placed in the anterior region. Other parameters, such as as gingival (GI) and plaque (PI) indexes in different EA groups, were considered as secondary outcomes. The authors hypothesized that with a straight-to-concave prosthetic emergence profile, EA ≥ 30° may not significantly influence peri-implant soft tissue measurements if compared to values of EA < 30°.

2. Materials and Methods

2.1. Patient Selection

The present retrospective evaluation was conducted in accordance with the fundamental principles of the Helsinki Declaration. Ethical Committee agreement (Prot. No. EC 02.04.20 REF 28/20) was obtained to complete the clinical measurement procedures mentioned below. The STROBE (Strengthening the Reporting of Observational Studies in

Epidemiology, strobe-statement.org (accessed on 2 February 2014)) guideline checklist of items was followed.

Patients needing an implant-supported fixed rehabilitation in anterior areas were included; the same implant system was used (Anyridge, MegaGen Implant Co., Gyeongbuk, Korea) from 2014 to 2017; clinical parameters and EA measurements were assessed.

Moreover, restorations with concave emergence profile (EP) at buccal aspect were included in order to not negatively interfere with all the different components of the transition zone (Figure 2), especially the biological boundary area [14]. The EP, corresponding to the restoration contour as per the definition of the Glossary of Prosthodontic Terms GTP-9 [8], was classified as concave, straight and convex on the buccal aspect during the digital EA measurement procedures.

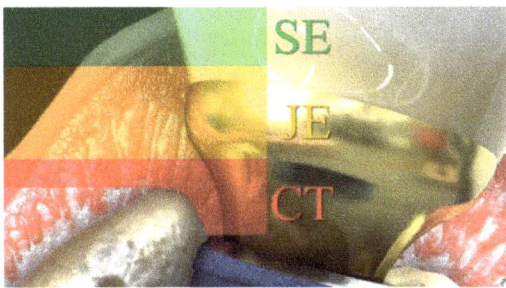

Figure 2. Sagittal section of the supracrestal soft tissues around implants and corresponding prosthetic components: connective tissues CT (red area), junctional epithelium JE (yellow area) and sulcular epithelium SE (green area), respectively.

Written consent about the study objectives was signed by the patients. Patients with single or multiple gaps were included and followed for a period of 3 years.

Patients with severe clenching or bruxism, systemic diseases, a history of radiation therapy in the head and neck region, inadequate compliance, and who were smokers (more than 15 cigarettes per day) were excluded.

The following additional data were collected: implant features as diameter and length, prosthesis type, implant site, date of prosthetic delivery.

2.2. Surgical and Prosthetic Procedures

As previously described by Lops et al. [10] a submerged healing technique was chosen for the implants that were placed (Anyridge, Megagen Implants, Seoul, Korea) 1 to 2 mm below the crestal level [15], as recommended by the manufacturer.

Distances of at least 3 mm, and from 1.5 to 3 mm, were chosen between implants, and between an implant and the adjacent tooth [16–19], respectively.

Only restorations from the premolar to the contralateral area were considered: fixed single crown (SC) and partial fixed prosthesis (FPD) were considered, respectively. For cemented restorations, abutments were torqued down to 25 Ncm and a temporary cement (Temp-Bond Clear, Kerr Corporation, Orange, CA, USA) was used. Differently, a torque of 25 Ncm was used to secure screw-retained prostheses.

2.3. Clinical and Digital Evaluations

Probing pocket depth (PPD), plaque index (PI) and gingival index (GI) [20–23] were assessed with a calibrated plastic probe (TPS probe, Vivadent, Schaan, Liechtenstein). Four sites for each implant (mesial, distal, buccal and lingual) were considered for recording probing depth scores.

GI scores ranged from 0 to 3 (0 = normal gingiva; 1 = mild inflammation: slight change in color, slight oedema. No bleeding on probing; 2 = moderate inflammation: redness, oedema and glazing. Bleeding on probing; 3 = severe inflammation: marked redness and oedema. Ulceration. Tendency to spontaneous bleeding).

Similarly, PI scores ranged from 0 to 3, respectively (0 = no plaque in the gingival area; 1 = a film of plaque adhering to the free gingival margin and adjacent area of the tooth. The plaque may only be recognized by running a probe across the tooth surface; 2 = moderate accumulation of soft deposits within the gingival pocket, on the gingival margin and/or adjacent tooth surface, which can be seen by the naked eye; 3 = abundance of soft matter within the gingival pocket and/or on the gingival margin and adjacent tooth surface).

Additionally, for GI and PI, indexes were calculated. The aforementioned parameters were recorded at 3 years of follow-up for each implant included in the present report.

The angle between the tangent of the transitional contour relative to the long axis of the implant was defined as the emergence angle (EA) by following the GTP-9 indications [8]. The angle assessment was digitally performed after turning every plaster master cast into a digital form, and using the digital restoration model as a reference for the EA measurements. The buccal aspect of the restoration was used for EA calculation (Figure 3).

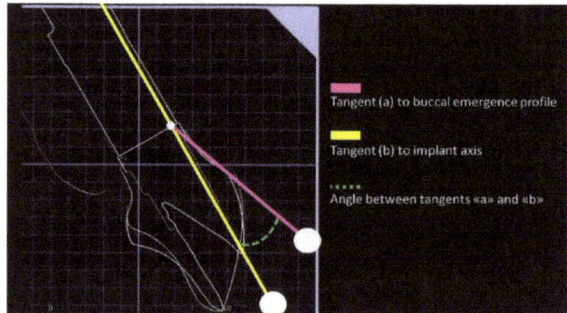

Figure 3. Emergence angle (EA) calculation procedure. After turning the analogic impression into a digital form, the customized emergence profile shape was planned and designed. The EA was calculated by drawing a line (yellow) parallel to the implant axis, and a pink line from the implant to the abutment connection point to the emergence profile. The angle of the intersection between pink and yellow lines resulted in the emergence angle (EA). If EA score was ≥30 degrees, the restoration was allocated to Group 1, while if it was <30 degrees the restoration was allocated to Group 2.

The definitive restoration EA angle was used for the group allocation (Figure 4).

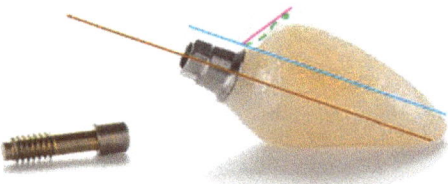

Figure 4. Emergence angle (EA) definition. Brown line: parallel to implant long axis. Blue line: parallel to the brown line and the line tangential to the implant shoulder. Pink line: from implant to abutment connection point to the emergence profile. The angle of the intersection between pink and blue lines resulted in the emergence angle (EA). Green line: buccal emergence profile (EP) shape. A concave area provides a support to the junctional epithelium, while the convex area supports the sulcular epithelium.

Group 1 EA ≥ 30°, Group 2 EA < 30° (Figure 5).

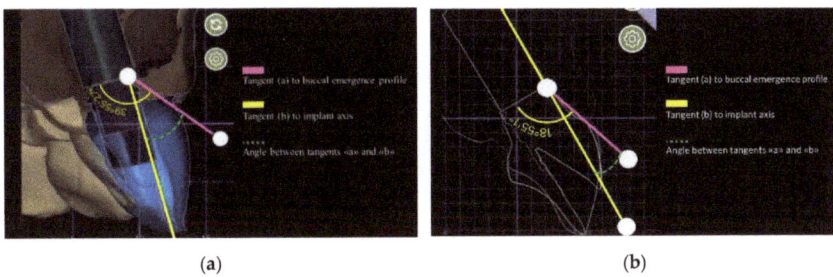

(a) (b)

Figure 5. (**a**) Emergence angle (EA) calculation procedure. An EA score ≥30 degrees allocated the restoration to Group 1; (**b**) Emergence angle (EA) calculation procedure. An EA score <30 degrees allocated the restoration to Group 2.

The transmucosal abutment was considered as a part of restoration. The shape and emergence angle (EA) of each prosthesis was selected by the dental technician depending on the specific features of the edentulous site to be restored. Measurements were repeated twice by the same operator (LV), and intra-operator reliability was calculated.

2.4. Statistical Analysis

Data were collected at site level. Quantitative variables were described using mean and standard deviation while categorical variables were summarized as counts and percentages. PPD was modelled at site level using a linear mixed model (LMM), with random intercept, in order to account for within-patient data clustering. Similarly, both PI and GI (coded 0 or greater than 0), considered as binary outcomes at site level and nested within the patient, were modelled using generalized linear mixed models (GLMM) assuming a binomial family distribution. Results are reported as estimates and corresponding 95% confidence intervals. All tests were two-sided and assumed a 5% significance level. All analyses were performed using "R project" statistical computing and graphics software (version 4.2.1, https://www.r-project.org (accessed on 23 April 2022)).

3. Results

Fifty-seven patients (24 males and 33 females, respectively), aged from 24 to 74 years (mean age 51.2 ± 27.2 years), treated with a total of 220 implants, and followed in a 3-year period from the definitive prosthesis installation, were included in the present study. Implant length is reported in Tables 1 and 2. Fixture distribution by implant site is reported in Table 3.

Table 1. Distribution of implant length in Group 1 (EA ≥ 30°) and Group 2 (EA < 30°).

		Group 1	Group 2	Total
Implant Length (mm)	7	3 (2%)	1 (1.5%)	4 (2%)
	8.5	4 (3%)	1 (1.5%)	5 (2%)
	10	20 (13%)	6 (9%)	26 (12%)
	11.5	2 (1%)	8 (12%)	10 (5%)
	13	100 (65%)	41 (61%)	141 (64%)
	15	24 (16%)	10 (15%)	34 (15%)
Total		153	67	220

Table 2. Frequency of implant diameter in Group 1 (EA ≥ 30°) and Group 2 (EA < 30°).

		Group 1	Group 2	Total
Implant Diameter (mm)	3.5	38 (25%)	25 (37%)	63 (29%)
	4.0	69 (45%)	23 (34%)	92 (42%)
	4.5	43 (28%)	19 (28%)	62 (28%)
	5.0	1 (0.6%)	0 (0%)	1 (0.4%)
	5.5	1 (0.6%)	0 (0%)	1 (0.4%)
	6.5	1 (0.6%)	0 (0%)	1 (0.4%)
Total		153	67	220

Table 3. Frequency of implant distribution by implant site in Group 1 and Group 2.

		Group 1	Group 2	Total
Implant Placement region	Incisor and Canine	56 (37%)	36 (54%)	92 (42%)
	Premolar	97 (63%)	31 (46%)	128 (58%)
Total		153	67	220
Upper or Lower Jaw	Mandible	98 (64%)	30 (45%)	128 (58%)
	Maxilla	55 (36%)	37 (55%)	92 (42%)
Total		153	67	220

Furthermore, a descriptive analysis of gender, systemic diseases and smoking habit distribution for the different EA groups is reported in Table 4. Distribution of prosthesis type was as follows: 34 SC: single crown; 62 FPD: fixed partial denture. The mean restorations EA in Groups 1 and 2 was 46.4 ± 12.2 and 24.5 ± 4.7 degrees, respectively. A mean PPD of 1.86 ± 0.35 mm and 1.81 ± 0.33 mm were found, respectively, in Group 1 and 2 (Table 5).

Table 4. Gender, systemic diseases and smoking habit distribution of Group 1 (EA ≥ 30°) and Group 2 (EA < 30°) patients.

		Group 1	Group 2	Total
Gender	F	82 (54%)	43 (64%)	125 (57%)
	M	71 (46%)	24 (36%)	95 (43%)
Total		153	67	220
Systemic diseases & smoking habit	Diabetes	12 (8%)	6 (9%)	18 (8%)
	Bisphosphonate ex-consumers	1 (0.6%)	0 (0%)	1 (0.4%)
	Smokers	35 (23%)	10 (15%)	45 (20%)
	Non-smokers and no systemic diseases	105 (69%)	51 (76%)	156 (71%)
Total		153	67	220

Table 5. Probing pocket depth in Group 1 (EA ≥ 30°) and Group 2 (EA < 30°).

		Group 1	Group 2	Overall
PPD	Mean (SD)	1.86 (0.35)	1.81 (0.33)	1.85 (0.34)
	Median (IQR)	2.00 (0.33)	2.00 (0.33)	2.00 (0.33)

A PPD difference of 0.062 mm was calculated between the two groups and was not statistically significant ($p = 0.237$). No statistical difference emerged when considering the implant site when the values of Groups 1 and 2 were compared (Table 6).

Table 6. *Linear mixed models* for PPD parameter.

Group Comparison		Sup/Inf	Ant/Post	Difference	Lower.CL	Upper.CL	p Value
Group 1	Group 2	Sup	Ant	0.166	−0.010	0.342	0.06484986
Group 1	Group 2	Inf	Ant	0.068	−0.115	0.252	0.46485740
Group 1	Group 2	Sup	Post	0.078	−0.103	0.260	0.39443006
Group 1	Group 2	Inf	Post	−0.019	−0.193	0.155	0.82867473
Group Comparison				Difference	Lower.CL	Upper.CL	p Value
Group 1 (≥30°)	Group 2 (<30°)			0.062	−0.041	0.164	0.2379016

The PI index in the two groups was scored as positive in 82 and 87% of implants, respectively, for Groups 1 and 2. On the whole, 184 (84%) of the 220 sites were scored as positive after 3 years of follow-up (Table 7). The difference between the two groups was not statistically significant ($p = 0.599$). Furthermore, no statistical difference of positive values was shown considering the implant site when the values of Groups 1 and 2 were compared (Table 8). GI index in the two groups was scored as 0 in 94 and 93% of implants, respectively, for Groups 1 and 2 (Table 9). Profuse bleeding at probing was diagnosed nine (5.9%) and five times (7.5%) for Groups 1 and 2, respectively. Such difference was not statistically significant ($p = 0.76$).

Table 7. Plaque index in Group 1 (EA ≥ 30°) and Group 2 (EA < 30°).

		Group 1	Group 2	Total
PI	Positive (from 1 to 3)	126 (82%)	58 (87%)	184 (84%)
	Negative (0)	27 (18%)	9 (13%)	36 (16%)
	Total	153	67	220

Table 8. *Linear mixed models* for PI parameter.

Group Comparison		Sup/Inf	Ant/Post	OR	Asymp.LCL	Asymp.UCL	p Value
Group 1	Group 2	Sup	Ant	1.273	0.269	6.024	0.7610423
Group 1	Group 2	Inf	Ant	0.803	0.162	3.976	0.7884486
Group 1	Group 2	Sup	Post	0.707	0.121	4.143	0.7003673
Group 1	Group 2	Inf	Post	0.446	0.083	2.395	0.3463866
Group Comparison				OR	Asymp.LCL	Asymp.UCL	p Value
Group 1 (≥30°)	Group 2 (<30°)			0.778	0.305	1.984	0.5991774

Table 9. Gingival index in Group 1 (EA ≥ 30°) and Group 2 (EA < 30°).

		Group 1	Group 2	Total
GI	0	144 (94%)	62 (93%)	206 (94%)
	1	0 (0%)	0 (0%)	0 (0%)
	2	5 (3%)	2 (3%)	7 (3%)
	3	4 (3%)	3 (4%)	7 (3%)
Total		153	67	220

4. Discussion

Final implant-supported restoration contour is crucial to achieve esthetic outcome (Figures 6–8). Different transition zone areas were identified with different features [14] and described as the 1 mm subgingival area apical to the free gingival margin. This so-called esthetic area should be convex in order to properly support the free gingival margin, and its shape is directly correlated to the buccal-to-palatal implant inclination. Secondly, a boundary area apical to the esthetic zone measures approximately 1–2 mm and should be concave in order to leave proper space for the soft tissues. The implant position and the choice of the restoration prosthetic components may interfere with the soft tissue thickness and the stability of apical-to-coronal transition zone dimensions. More apical and directly coronal to the implant-to-abutment connection area is 1–1.5 mm of connective tissue related to the peri-implant bone stability. The vertical dimension of such space is dependent on the implant design and the crestal or sub-crestal implant placement.

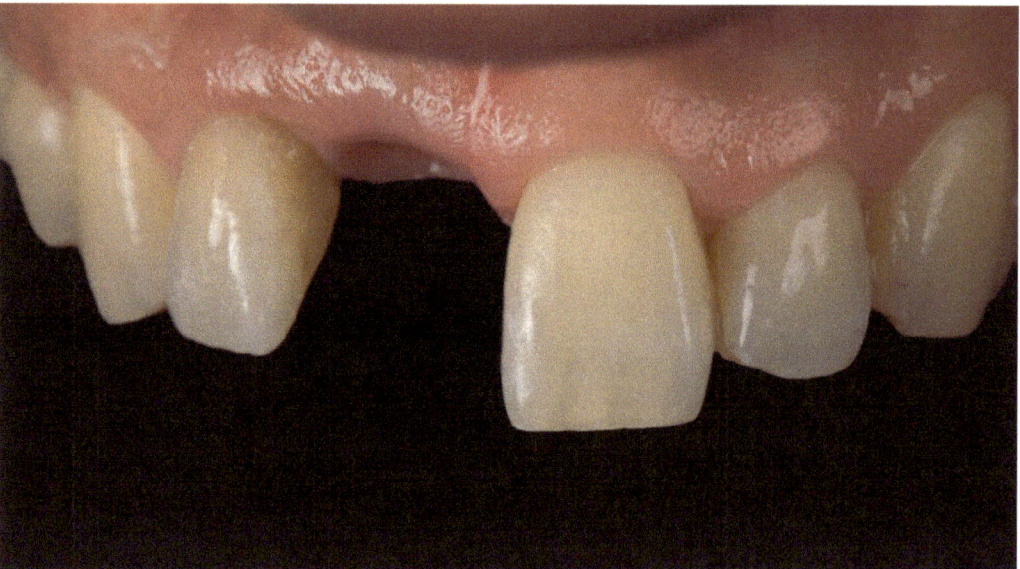

Figure 6. Stable peri-implant soft tissues before screwing the implant-supported restoration. Frontal view.

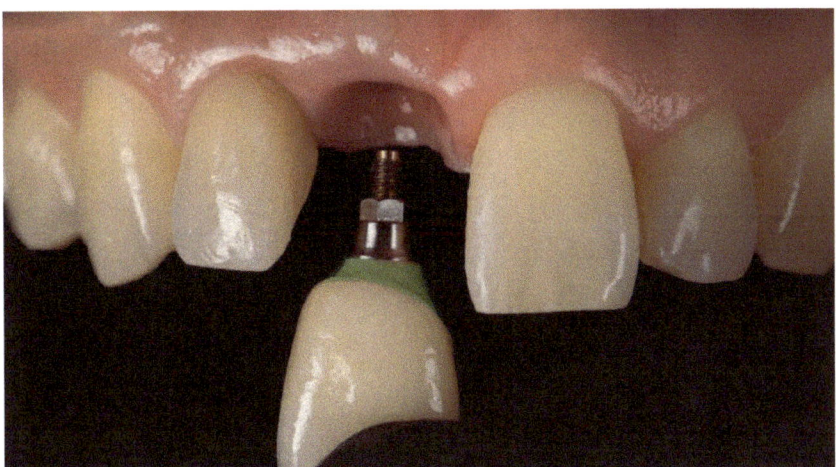

Figure 7. The restoration area marked in green will face peri-implant soft tissues from the junctional to the sulcular epithelium areas, respectively. Frontal view.

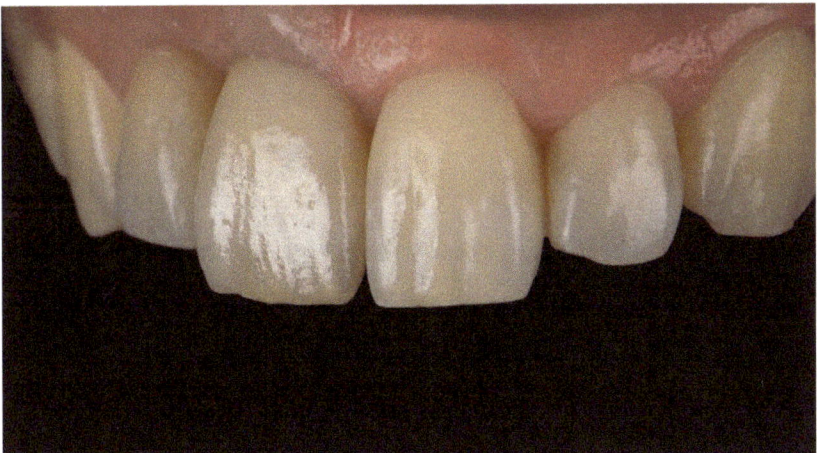

Figure 8. Implant-supported restoration in place.

Even though such transition zone areas are actually well known and the geometry of prosthetic restoration is accepted, there is no clear quantitative measurement of the parameters related to a proper prosthetic profile contour. The emergence profile and angle concepts were used to describe of such circumscribed soft tissues. As reported by the ninth edition of the Glossary of Prosthodontic Terms [8], the "emergence profile" (EP) and "emergence angle" (EA) are described similarly for both natural teeth and implant prostheses; however, extrapolating these terms on implant prostheses, EP is defined as the restoration contour, including the abutment and crown complex. Differently, EA is defined as the angle of an implant restoration transitional contour as determined by the relation of the surface of the abutment to the long axis of the implant body.

In the present study, ≥30 and <30° EA were investigated in two groups of implant-supported reconstructions, respectively. All implants were restored by means of a 5° internal conical connection and a platform shifting of the prosthetic abutments from the fixture diameter. Such feature, related to the implant-to-abutment connection, seems to be effective in the maintenance of peri-implant bone stability in the mid-to-long term [10]. After 3 years of follow-up, EA digitally measured on the buccal side was correlated to peri-implant soft tissue parameters as PPD, PI and GI indexes, respectively. No significant differences between the two groups were found for each parameter investigated. Such finding shows that the EA parameter may not itself affect peri-implant soft tissue stability, but only if related to a specific emergence profile shape; in a cross-sectional study by Yi et al., the influence of prosthetic features was investigated through a comprehensive analysis with other known risk factors. EA had a significant effect on the prevalence of peri-implantitis only if associated with a straight or convex EP [24]. On the contrary, if it was associated with a concave emergence profile, EA was not related to an increased peri-implantitis rate. These outcomes perfectly agree with those of the present paper, with EA measured at the buccal aspect of the transition zone. A similar conclusion was also reported by other authors when EA was measured at the inter-proximal aspect: in a cross-sectional radiographic analysis by Katafuchi et al. [12], the highest peri-implantitis rate (37.8%) was observed only if the restoration emergence was combined with a convex profile. Similar outcomes were found in a retrospective analysis by Lops et al. [10]: marginal bone loss and plaque indexes were not statistically different with interproximal EA > and $\leq$30 degrees after 3 years of follow-up. The EP in all the restorations were straight or concave. Even in the similar conclusions by Katafuchi et al. [12] and Lops et al. [10], a different method was used to assess EA parameters in the present report; in fact, not a radiographic but a digital workflow was followed to investigate buccal EA.

From a clinical point of view, the present study outcomes may lead to the conclusion that EA > 30 degrees can be chosen to plan implant-supported reconstructions with high esthetic impact without an increase of peri-implant disease risk, as long as a concave EP and a stable implant-to-abutment connection is provided. Even then, access to oral hygiene procedures should be guaranteed to avoid the risk of peri-implant disease [13,24–26] by avoiding prosthesis buccal over-contouring in the esthetic area. Nevertheless, more prospective and long-term data are required to confirm this trend.

5. Conclusions

Peri-implant soft-tissue stability does not seem to be influenced by EA itself when a correct emergence profile is provided for implant supported reconstructions in anterior areas, even if this parameter is more than 30 degrees.

Author Contributions: Conceptualization, D.L. and M.M.; validation, S.C., S.S. and E.R.; formal analysis, A.P.; investigation, S.C.; data curation, A.P. and L.V.; writing—original draft preparation, D.L. and L.V.; writing—review and editing, D.L. and B.B.; supervision, D.L. All authors have read and agreed to the published version of the manuscript.

Funding: This research received no external funding.

Institutional Review Board Statement: The study was conducted in accordance with the Declaration of Helsinki, and approved by the Institutional Review Board (or Ethics Committee) of UNIVERSITY OF MILAN (Prot. No. EC 02.04.20 REF 28/20).

Informed Consent Statement: Informed consent was obtained from all subjects involved in the study.

Data Availability Statement: The data presented in this study are available on request from the corresponding author. The data are not publicly available due to privacy policies.

Conflicts of Interest: The authors declare no conflict of interest.

References

1. Linkevicius, T.; Puisys, A. Crestal bone stability around implants with horizontally matching connection after soft tissue thickening: A prospective clinical trial. *Clin. Implant Dent. Relat. Res.* **2015**, *17*, 497–508. [CrossRef] [PubMed]
2. Kim, S.; Oh, K. Influence of transmucosal designs of three one-piece implant systems on early tissue responses: A histometric study in beagle dogs. *Int. J. Oral. Maxillofac. Implant.* **2010**, *25*, 309–314.

3. Kaddas, C.; Papamanoli, E. Etiology and Treatment of Peri-Implant Soft Tissue Dehiscences: A Narrative Review. *Dent. J.* **2022**, *10*, 86. [CrossRef] [PubMed]
4. Lin, G.; Chan, H. The significance of keratinized mucosa on implant health: A systematic review. *J. Periodontol.* **2013**, *84*, 1755–1767. [CrossRef]
5. Cinquini, C.; Marchio, V. Histologic Evaluation of Soft Tissues around Dental Implant Abutments: A Narrative Review. *Materials* **2022**, *15*, 3811. [CrossRef]
6. Schoenbaum, T.R. Abutment emergence profile and its effect on Peri-implant tissues. *Compend Contin Educ. Dent.* **2015**, *36*, 474–479.
7. Gonzalez-Martin, O.; Lee, E. Contour Management of Implant Restorations for optimal emergence profiles: Guidelines for immediate and delayed provisional restorations. *Int. J. Periodontics Restor. Dent.* **2020**, *40*, 61–70. [CrossRef] [PubMed]
8. Ferro, K.J.; Morgano, S.M.; Driscoll, C.F.; Freilich, M.A.; Guckes, A.D.; Knoernschild, K.L.; Twain, M. The glossary of prosthodontic terms: Ninth edition. *J. Prosthet. Dent.* **2017**, *117*, 1–105.
9. Su, H.; Gonzalez-Martin, O. Considerations of implant abutment and crown contour: Critical contour and subcritical contour. *Int. J. Periodontics Restor. Dent.* **2010**, *30*, 335–343.
10. Lops, D.; Romeo, E. Marginal bone maintenance and different prosthetic emergence angles. A 3-years prospective study. *J. Clin. Med.* **2022**, *11*, 2014. [CrossRef] [PubMed]
11. Sanz, M.; Lang, N.P. Seventh European Workshop on Periodontology of the European Academy of Periodontology at the Parador at la Granja, Segovia, Spain. *J. Clin. Periodontol.* **2011**, *38*, 1–2. [CrossRef]
12. Katafuchi, M.; Weinstein, B.F. Restoration contour is a risk indicator for peri-implantitis: A cross-sectional radiographic analysis. *J. Clin. Periodontol.* **2018**, *45*, 225–232. [CrossRef] [PubMed]
13. Mattheos, N.; Janda, M. Impact of design elements of the implant supracrestal complex (ISC) on the risk of peri- implant mucositis and peri-implantitis: A critical review. *Clin. Oral. Implant. Res.* **2021**, *32*, 181–202. [CrossRef]
14. Gomez-Meda, R.; Esquivel, J. The esthetic biological contour concept for implant restoration emergence profile design. *Int. J. Esthet. Restor. Dent.* **2021**, *33*, 173–184. [CrossRef] [PubMed]
15. Lops, D.; Stocchero, M. Degree Internal Conical Connection and Marginal Bone Stability around Subcrestal Implants: A Retrospective Analysis. *Materials* **2020**, *13*, 3123. [CrossRef] [PubMed]
16. Cosyn, J.; Eghbali, A. Immediate single-tooth implants in the anterior maxilla: 3-year results of a case series on hard and soft tissue response and aesthetics. *J. Clin. Periodontol.* **2011**, *38*, 746–753. [CrossRef] [PubMed]
17. Galindo-Moreno, P.; Fernández-Jiménez, A. Influence of the crown-implant connection on the preservation of peri-implant bone: A retrospective multifactorial analysis. *J. Oral. Maxillofacc. Surg.* **2015**, *30*, 384–390. [CrossRef]
18. Lops, D.; Chiapasco, M. Incidence of inter-proximal papilla between a tooth and an adjacent immediate implant placed into a fresh extraction socket: 1-year prospective study. *Clin. Oral. Implant. Res.* **2008**, *19*, 1135–1140. [CrossRef]
19. Lops, D.; Parpaiola, A. Interproximal Papilla Stability Around CAD/CAM and Stock Abutments in Anterior Regions: A 2-Year Prospective Multicenter Cohort Study. *Int. J. Periodontics Restor. Dent.* **2017**, *37*, 657–665. [CrossRef] [PubMed]
20. McClanahan, S.; Bartizek, R. Identification and consequences of distinct Löe-Silness gingival index examiner styles for the clinical assessment of gingivitis. *J. Periodontol.* **2001**, *72*, 383–392. [CrossRef] [PubMed]
21. Löe, H. The Gingival Index, the Plaque Index and the Retention Index Systems. *J. Periodontol.* **1967**, *38*, 610–616. [CrossRef]
22. Mombelli, A.; Lang, N.P. Clinical parameters for evalutation of dental implants. *Periodontol 2000* **1994**, *4*, 81–86. [CrossRef] [PubMed]
23. Mombelli, A.; Lang, N.P. The diagnosis and treatment of peri-implantitis. *Periodontol 2000* **1998**, *16*, 575–579. [CrossRef] [PubMed]
24. Yi, Y.; Koo, K. Association of prosthetic features and peri-implantitis: A cross sectional study. *J. Clin. Periodontol.* **2020**, *47*, 392–403. [CrossRef] [PubMed]
25. Serino, G.; Ström, C. Peri-implantitis in partially edentulous patients: Association with inadequate plaque control. *Clin. Oral. Implant. Res.* **2009**, *20*, 169–174. [CrossRef] [PubMed]
26. De Tapia, B.; Mozas, C. Adjunctive effect of modifying the implant-supported prosthesis in the treatment of peri-implant peri-implant mucositis. *J. Clin. Periodontol.* **2019**, *46*, 1050–1060. [CrossRef] [PubMed]

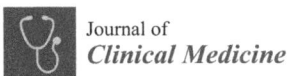

Article

Intraoral Scanning as an Alternative to Evaluate the Accuracy of Dental Implant Placements in Partially Edentate Situations: A Prospective Clinical Case Series

Jan van Hooft [1,*,†], Guido Kielenstijn [1,*,†], Jeroen Liebregts [2], Frank Baan [3], Gert Meijer [2], Jan D'haese [1], Ewald Bronkhorst [1] and Luc Verhamme [3]

1 Department of Dentistry, Radboudumc Nijmegen, Philips van Leydenlaan 25, 6525 EX Nijmegen, The Netherlands
2 Department of Oral and Maxillofacial Surgery, Radboudumc Nijmegen, Geert Grooteplein Zuid 10, 6525 GA Nijmegen, The Netherlands
3 3D Lab, Radboudumc Nijmegen, Geert Grooteplein Zuid 10, 6525 GA Nijmegen, The Netherlands
* Correspondence: jan.cm.vanhooft@radboudumc.nl (J.v.H.); guidentistry@outlook.com (G.K.)
† These authors contributed equally to this work.

Abstract: (1) Background: For years, Cone-Beam Computed Tomography's (CBCT) have been the golden standard to evaluate implant placement accuracy. By validating Intraoral Scans (IOS) as an alternative to determine implant placement accuracy, a second CBCT could be avoided. (2) Methods: Using dynamic guided implant surgery, 23 implants were placed in 16 partially edentate patients. Preoperatively, both CBCT and IOS (Trios® 3) were obtained and subsequently imported into DTX Studio™ planning software to determine the ideal implant location. A CBCT scan and an IOS including scan abutments were acquired immediately after placement. Both postoperative CBCT and postoperative IOS were used to compare the achieved implant position with the planned implant position and were projected and analyzed using the Implant Position Orthogonal Projection (IPOP) method. (3) Results: Mean differences between the CBCT and IOS methods on the mesio–distal plane were 0.09 mm ($p = 0.419$) at the tip, 0.01 mm ($p = 0.910$) at the shoulder, $-0.55°$ ($p = 0.273$) in angulation, and 0.2 mm ($p = 0.280$) in implant depth. Mean differences between both methods on the bucco-lingual/bucco-palatal plane were 0.25 mm ($p = 0.000$) at the tip, 0.12 mm ($p = 0.011$) at the shoulder, $-0.81°$ ($p = 0.002$) in angulation, and 0.17 mm ($p = 0.372$) in implant depth. A statistical analysis was performed using a paired t-test. All mesiodistal deviations between the two methods showed no significant differences ($p > 0.05$). Buccolingual/buccopalatal deviations showed no significant difference in implant depth deviation. However, significant differences were found at the tip, shoulder, and angulation ($p < 0.05$). These values are of minimal clinical significance. (4) Conclusions: This study supports the hypothesis that a postoperative IOS is a valid alternative for determining implant placement accuracy.

Keywords: oral implantology; intraoral scan; accuracy; cone-beam computed tomography; oral surgery

1. Introduction

When osseointegrated implants became introduced in dentistry, their primary role was to re-establish a loss of function. Later on, due to constant advancements in implant design, ameliorated implant surfaces, and the introduction of challenging treatment protocols, aesthetic demands became more relevant. Patients insisted on shorter treatment protocols with predictable results both from a functional and esthetical viewpoint. With these increasing demands and expectations, the role of preoperative implant planning also becomes more relevant.

Almost 25 years ago, computer-aided design and manufacturing was introduced in implant dentistry as a tool to enhance accuracy and precision to install dental implants.

Citation: van Hooft, J.; Kielenstijn, G.; Liebregts, J.; Baan, F.; Meijer, G.; D'haese, J.; Bronkhorst, E.; Verhamme, L. Intraoral Scanning as an Alternative to Evaluate the Accuracy of Dental Implant Placements in Partially Edentate Situations: A Prospective Clinical Case Series. J. Clin. Med. 2022, 11, 5876. https://doi.org/10.3390/jcm11195876

Academic Editors: Adolfo Di Fiore and Giulia Brunello

Received: 16 August 2022
Accepted: 29 September 2022
Published: 5 October 2022

Publisher's Note: MDPI stays neutral with regard to jurisdictional claims in published maps and institutional affiliations.

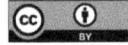

Copyright: © 2022 by the authors. Licensee MDPI, Basel, Switzerland. This article is an open access article distributed under the terms and conditions of the Creative Commons Attribution (CC BY) license (https://creativecommons.org/licenses/by/4.0/).

Currently, there are two pathways to implement this technology in clinical practice. One can either use a static approach using preprinted surgical templates or opt for dynamic guided surgery, which is also known as navigation surgery. The last one, which is the most recently developed, is based on motion-tracking technology. It enables the real-time visualization of both drills and fixture on the combined image of the preoperative Cone-Beam Computed Tomography (CBCT) and intraoral scan (IOS), where the planned location is also visible [1].

To evaluate the accuracy of implant installation, the gold standard is to make use of a postoperative CBCT [2,3]. Applying voxel-based matching [4,5], both pre- and postoperative CBCT are aligned on top of each other to measure the deviation between the actual position of the dental implants and their pre-surgical position in the planning software.

In recent years, the IOS was introduced in dental practices as a valid alternative for conventional impression protocols. To determine implant placement accuracy, a postoperative IOS could be a viable alternative to a postoperative CBCT. In this manner, the radiation load for patients is reduced by avoiding a postoperative CBCT and the associated radiation dose of 2 to 1000µSv (equivalent of 2 to 200 panoramic radiographs) [6].

Besides the IOS, there are other, non-invasive methods for determining implant placement accuracy. The photogrammetric method [7] can determine the implant's location using photographs from multiple angles, and the implant is made of a cast from the patient's jaw.

Another method is the contact scan method, where, by also using a postoperative cast of the patient's jaw, the location of the placed implant is determined using a contact scanner.

However, both methods require extra steps, since, in a digital workflow, an IOS is necessary anyway to fabricate the dental prosthesis, and a (plaster) cast of the patient's jaw is normally not necessary; moreover, these methods also require either dedicated cameras or a contact scanner, which are both not needed for regular treatment protocols.

The aim of this prospective clinical case series was to evaluate if a postoperative IOS is a reliable alternative to a postoperative CBCT to determine dental implant placement accuracy in an in vivo setting and to describe deviations between both methods.

2. Materials and Methods

2.1. Patient Selection

In total, 16 dentate patients, referred to the department of Oral and Maxillofacial Surgery at Radboudumc Nijmegen to install at least one dental implant, were enrolled in this study. Patients were excluded if they were suffering from active periodontal disease, severe bruxism, or when intravenous bisphosphonates were administered. All patients provided written informed consent. Patients were not selected regarding implant location. They were treated according to their specific desire to restore the edentulous area. The protocol was evaluated and approved by the ethical committee of Oost-Nederland (file nr 2020-6449) and performed according to the Declaration of Helsinki.

2.2. Preoperative Data Acquisition

Prior to obtaining the preoperative CBCT scan (i-CAT® 3D Imaging System, Imaging Science International Inc, Hatfield, PA, USA), a small registration device, the x-clip (Nobel Biocare™, Zürich, Switzerland), with 3 metal reference points was placed on the teeth contralateral to the implant site. Subsequently, a CBCT scan was made with the x-clip 'in situ' (Figure 1) using a voxel size between 0.25 and 0.40 mm and a field of view of 6 cm × 6 cm. All images were exported and saved in DICOM (Digital Imaging and Communications in Medicine) format. To create an intraoral 3D model, an IOS (Trios® 3, 3Shape, Copenhagen, Denmark) was obtained, which was saved as a Standard Tessellation Language (STL) file. As such, additional information regarding soft tissues was acquired.

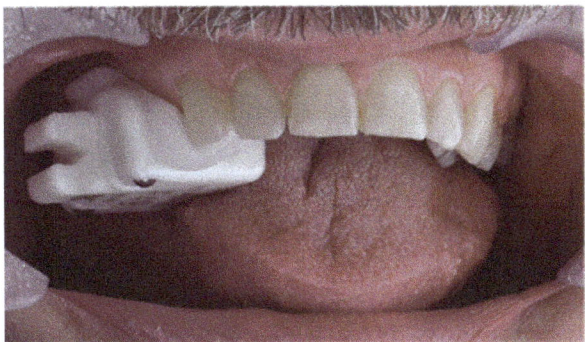

Figure 1. X-clip situated in the patient's mouth.

2.3. Virtual Implant Planning

Pre-op DICOM files and the IOS were uploaded in the DTX Studio™ (Nobel BioCare, Zürich, Switzerland) software (Figure 2) and subsequently matched automatically. In this software, the ideal implant location was determined, maintaining a safety margin relative to vital anatomical structures of 1.5 mm. XYZ coordinates for the planned implants tip and shoulder were obtained. Finally, virtual implant planning was imported into the X-guide® system (X-nav, Landsdale, PA, USA).

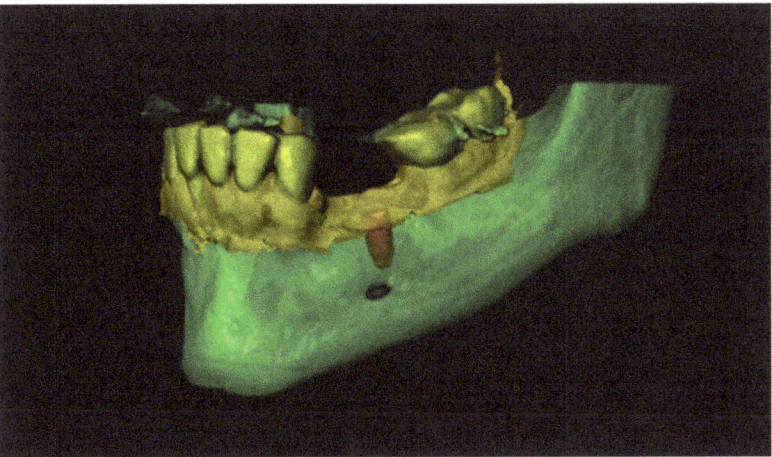

Figure 2. Virtual planning: green represents DICOM data, yellow represents the IOS data, and red represents the planned implant location.

2.4. Implant Placement

Surgery was performed under local anesthesia using appropriate aseptic and sterile protocols. During the entire procedure, the x-clip was fixed in the exact same location as during CBCT acquisition. Registration, calibration (Figure 3), and system checks were conducted before starting the surgery, as described in the X-Guide® manual. The X-Guide® uses the x-clip as a reference to determine the location of the implant drill as projected during preoperative planning. Osteotomies were prepared at a maximum of 1500 rpm and guided in real time by indicating the desired drilling pathway on the computer screen. An extra calibration process was completed preceding the use of each new drill. Prior to the preparation of the implant placement, no punching of the gingival tissues was performed. NobelParallel® Conical Connection (Nobel Biocare™, Zürich, Switzerland) implants or Nobel Active® (Nobel Biocare™, Zürich, Switzerland) implants were installed. All implants were placed by the same operator (J.L.), who was not involved in data collection and analysis.

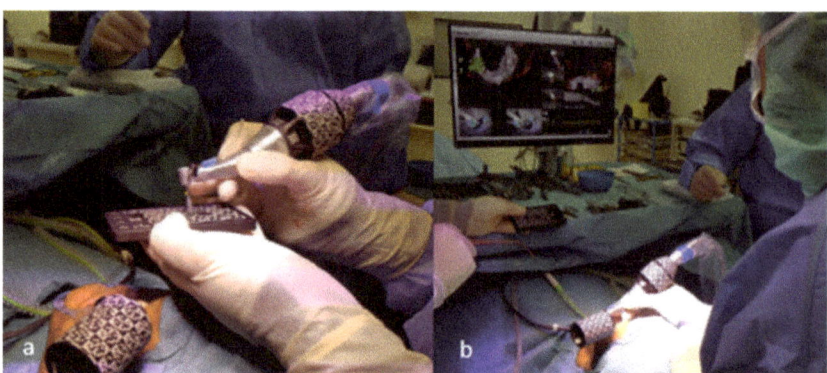

Figure 3. Calibration of the implant drill (**a**) and placement (**b**) of the implant using the X-Guide®.

2.5. Analysis of 3D Imaging Based on Postoperative CBCT and IOS

Immediately after the implant's placement, a scan abutment (Nobel Biocare, Zürich, Switzerland) was screwed onto the installed implants in order to obtain the postoperative IOS. Subsequently, the scan abutment was replaced with a healing abutment. A postoperative CBCT was obtained using the same settings and parameters as in the preoperative scans. Pre- and postoperative data (pre-op CBCT, post-op CBCT, pre-op IOS, and post-op IOS) were imported in the 3DMedX® software (v1.2.13.2, 3D Lab Radboudumc Nijmegen, The Netherlands) together with the planned implant location.

Pre- and postoperative CBCT images were matched using Voxel-Based Registration (VBR) [8]. Subsequently, a 3D model of the implant was segmented from the registered postoperative CBCT scan. Hereafter, a DICOM model of the implant (with the same diameter and length) was imported into the dataset and roughly aligned with the previously segmented postoperative implant model. After this initial alignment, a VBR procedure was applied to match the DICOM model of the implant accurately with the installed implant (Figure 4a–e).

To compare the postoperative IOS with the preoperative implant planning, first, a Surface-Based Registration (SBR) using the Iterative Closest Point (ICP) algorithm of the preoperative and postoperative IOS took place, based on the patient's own dentition as reference points excluding scan abutments. To visualize the implant on the postoperative IOS, a computer model, depicting the implant with the scan abutment on top, was loaded into 3DMedX®. SBR based on the scan abutment took place to import the implant model in the postoperative IOS. This resulted in a superimposition of the clinically placed implant over the virtually planned implant, as projected on the CBCT scan (Figure 5a–d).

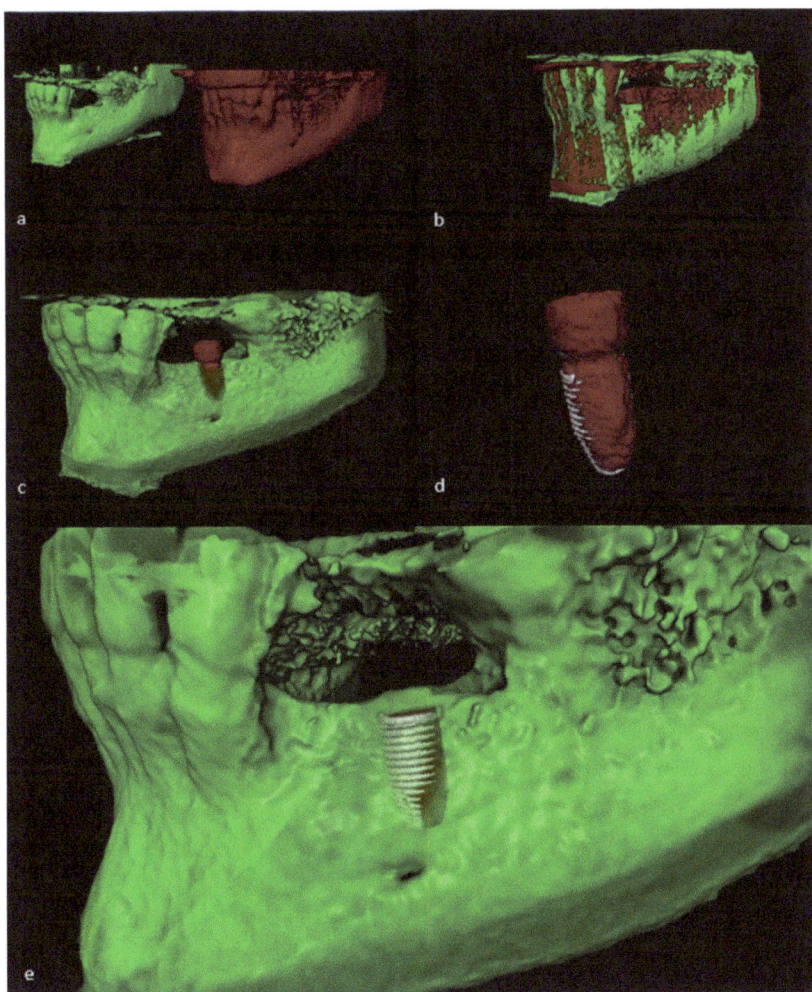

Figure 4. (**a–e**) The evaluation of the accuracy of implant placements based on postoperative CBCT. (**a**) 3D model derived from preoperative CBCT scan (green) and postoperative CBCT scan (red); (**b**) Voxel-based matching of the pre- and postoperative 3D model; (**c**) Segmented implant (red) of the postoperative 3D model; (**d**) Voxel-based matching of segmented implant and DICOM model implant (white); (**e**) 3D model of the jaw with the virtually planned implant (red) and the DICOM model corresponding with the placed implant (white).

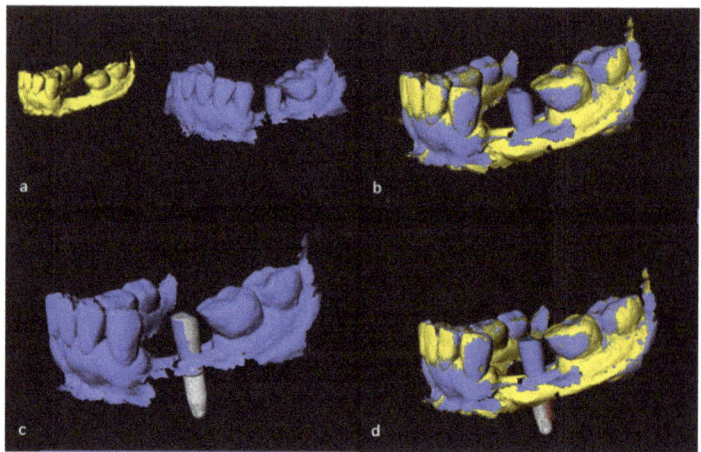

Figure 5. (**a–d**) Evaluation of accuracy of implant placement based on postoperative IOS. (**a**) Preoperative (yellow) and postoperative (blue) IOS 3D model; (**b**) Surface based registration of the pre- and postoperative 3D-model; (**c**) Surface based registration of implant model with scan-abutment (white); (**d**) 3D model of the jaw with planned (red) and placed (white) implant.

2.6. Implant Validation

After analyses and the matching of preoperative data with either the postoperative CBCT or the postoperative IOS, coordinates of the shoulder and tip of the placed implants were determined using 3DMedX® and MATLAB© (R2020b, The MathWorks, Inc., Natick, MA, USA) software. This resulted in two sets of x-, y-, and z-values, one set determined by means of postoperative IOS images and one set by means of postoperative CBCT images. Comparing these values with the coordinates of the planned implant position provided information on three aspects of implant placements, as displayed in Figure 6.

(a) Deviation in implant shoulder in millimeters (mm): three-dimensional distance between shoulder of planned and placed implant, measured from the axis;
(b) Deviation in implant tip in millimeters (mm): three-dimensional distance between tip of planned and placed implant, measured from the axis;
(c) Angular deviation in degrees (°): largest angle between the central, longitudinal axis of planned and realized implant positions.

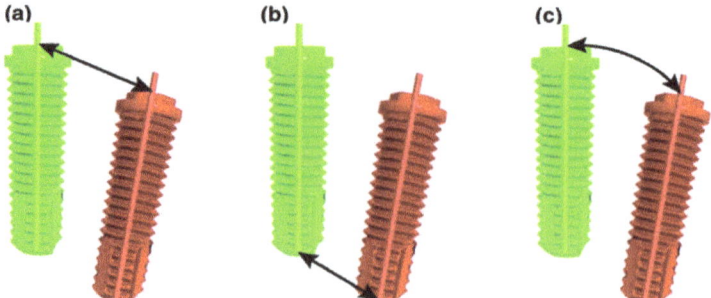

Figure 6. Implant placement deviations in 3D display: (**a**) deviation at the shoulder, (**b**) deviation at the tip, and (**c**) angular deviation.

Additionally, using the Implant Position Orthogonal Projection (IPOP) method, validated by Verhamme et al. [9], deviations were projected along the mesiodistal, buccolingual/palatal planes. To do so, six points were marked on the digital model of the dental arch, resulting in a curve corresponding with the dental arch. By means of both a plane perpendicular and a plane tangent to this arch at the place of the placed implant, information was obtained on the deviation of the implant's placement, as projected in the mesio–distal (MD) plane and the bucco-lingual/bucco-palatal (BL/BP) plane. This was performed for the data extracted from both the CBCT scan and IOS. By means of the IPOP method, deviations in implant depth on both planes were also determined:

2.7. Statistical Analysis

Statistical analysis of the data was performed using SPSS® software (v27, IBM Corp. Armonk, NY, USA). The differences between implant position determined by either CBCT scan or IOS were statistically analyzed using a paired t-test and were found significant if the p-value was <0.05:

3. Results

In total, 23 implants were placed in 16 patients (11 males and 5 females) with a mean age of 49 years (range 24–78 years). Nine patients received one implant for single-tooth replacement, six patients received two implants, both for single-tooth replacement, and one patient received two implants for an implant-supported bridge. Locations of all individual cases are displayed in Table 1. Deviations between planned and placed implants are displayed in Table 2. Mean deviations are based on absolute values.

Table 1. Implant location of all cases.

Case	Mandible/Maxilla	Implant Location
1	Maxilla	11
2	Mandible	36
3	Maxilla	15
4	Maxilla	16
5.1	Maxilla	13
5.2	Maxilla	12
6	Maxilla	21
7.1	Maxilla	12
7.2	Maxilla	14
8.1	Mandible	46
8.2	Mandible	47
9	Maxilla	12
10	Mandible	35
11.1	Maxilla	13
11.2	Maxilla	23
12.1	Mandible	36
12.2	Mandible	37
13	Maxilla	13
14.1	Maxilla	11
14.2	Maxilla	21
15.1	Maxilla	24
15.2	Maxilla	25
16	Maxilla	21

Table 2. Mean difference between planned and placed implants, as determined by CBCT and IOS.

		Mean (CBCT)	Standard Deviation (CBCT)	Mean (IOS)	Standard Deviation (CBCT)
Mesio-Distal plane	Tip (mm)	0.601	0.460	0.685	0.466
	Shoulder (mm)	0.473	0.350	0.486	0.348
	Angular (°)	1.643	1.220	2.288	1.608
	Depth (mm)	0.151	1.016	−0.045	0.692
Bucco-Lingual/Bucco-palatal plane	Tip (mm)	0.535	0.455	0.552	0.454
	Shoulder (mm)	0.500	0.489	0.549	0.451
	Angular (°)	1.755	1.555	1.421	1.169
	Depth (mm)	0.209	1.206	−0.045	0.680
3D plane	Tip (mm)	1.369	0.746	1.186	0.484
	Shoulder (mm)	1.265	0.773	1.057	0.429
	Angular (°)	2.625	1.494	2.835	1.595

Cone-Beam Computed Tomography (CBCT) and intraoral scan (IOS).

A paired t-test was performed and discrepancies between accuracy determinations by IOS and by CBCT were analyzed (Table 3). Before calculating discrepancies, mesial, lingual/palatal, and counterclockwise deviations were given a positive value, and distal, buccal, and clockwise deviations were labelled with a negative value. Boxplots of these deviations are displayed in Figures 7 and 8. To test whether the assumption that the small size of each cluster and the correlation between the measurement error between two different implants is weak, we repeated our analysis with multilevel regression analysis that allowed for clustering. This analysis virtually produced identical results.

Tip, shoulder, angular, and depth deviations, as projected on the MD plane and the depth deviation as projected on the BL/BP plane, were all statistically insignificant ($p > 0.05$). Tip, shoulder, and angular deviations as projected on the BL/BP plane were all statistically significant ($p < 0.05$). These deviations displayed a p-value of, respectively, 0.000, 0.011, and 0.002.

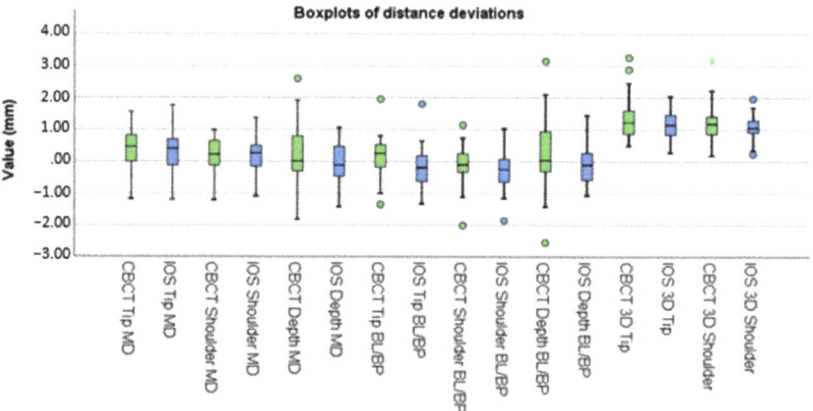

Figure 7. Boxplots of distance deviations.

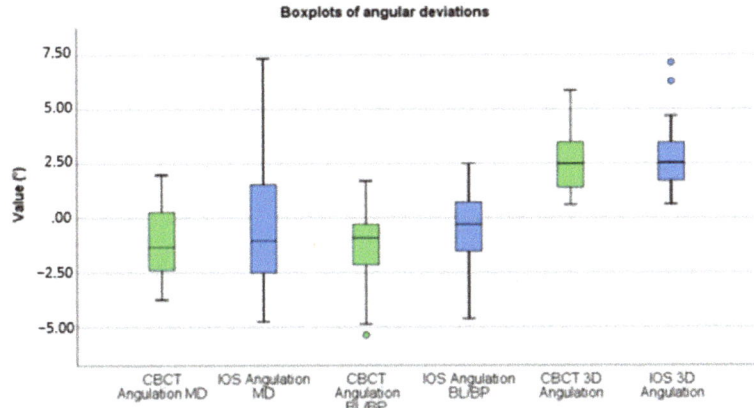

Figure 8. Boxplots of angular deviations.

Table 3. Statistical analysis of net deviations between CBCT and IOS.

		Mean	Standard Deviation	95% Confidence Interval of the Difference		p-Value
				Lower	Upper	
Mesio-Distal Plane	Tip (mm)	0.09	0.54	−0.14	0.33	0.419
	Shoulder (mm)	0.01	0.35	−0.14	0.16	0.910
	Angular (°)	−0.55	2.34	−1.56	0.46	0.273
	Depth	0.20	0.85	−0.17	0.57	0.280
Bucco-Lingual/Bucco-palatal plane	Tip (mm)	0.25	0.23	0.15	0.34	0.000 *
	Shoulder (mm)	0.12	0.20	0.03	0.21	0.011 *
	Angular (°)	−0.81	1.10	−1.28	−0.33	0.002 *
	Depth	0.17	0.88	−0.21	0.55	0.372

* Statistical significance.

4. Discussion

As computer-guided implant surgery was introduced in oral implantology, clinicians became aware of the relevance of accuracy. Generating a second, postoperative CBCT scan was previously the only possibility to evaluate implant placement accuracies. The introduction of IOS in dentistry led to the suggestion that an IOS could also be used to evaluate implant placements and thus avoids the need of a second postoperative CBCT scan.

CBCT and IOS validation methods displayed a mean absolute deviation, as compared to implant planning, of the implant shoulder in 3D orientation of, respectively, 1.27 and 1.06 mm; the implant tip displayed a deviation of, respectively, 1.37 and 1.19 mm and an angular deviation of, respectively, 2.63 and 2.84 degrees. This falls in line with the other recent literature regarding the implant placement accuracy of dynamic guided implant surgery [10–13].

To analyze deviations in 3D between IOS and CBCT scans, one could suffice with only calculating the differences between the achieved implant locations between these two imaging types. Since the direction of deviations is also clinically relevant, we focused on the difference between planned and achieved implant positions and, subsequently, defined the direction of the deviations by means of the IPOP method. Mesial, lingual/palatal, and counterclockwise deviations were given a positive value, implicating that distal, buccal, and clockwise deviations were labelled with a negative value. As a result, statistical analysis became feasible.

On the MD plane, no significant differences were found between validation with a postoperative IOS and CBCT scan. On the BL/BP plane, significant differences were found for tip deviations, shoulder deviations, and angular deviations. It concerns only minor differences of, respectively, 0.25 mm, 0.12 mm (both indicating that the IOS implant projection was more to the buccal side), and of −0.81° (the IOS implant projected a more counterclockwise rotation). One must keep in mind that deviations less than 0.25 mm are clinically irrelevant.

However, deviations larger than 1 mm are relevant indeed. One case displayed a discrepancy at the tip of 1.69 mm in MD direction and a difference in angulation of 6.26°. In this specific case, the postoperative IOS lacked information about soft tissues surrounding the scan abutment. Although the matching procedure on the scan abutment itself went well, in the end, this missing information led to a miscalculation by the IOS software with respect to the proper location of the scan abutment, as depicted in Figure 9. The matching of the IOS (light blue) and scan abutment DICOM model (grey) shows no errors at the left implant. However, the mesial implant, as segmented from the postoperative CBCT (yellow) and the corresponding DICOM implant model (white), does show a clear deviation between the CBCT model and the IOS model (green blue). This confirms that missing information relative to soft tissues indeed affects optimal matching for determining the implant's position.

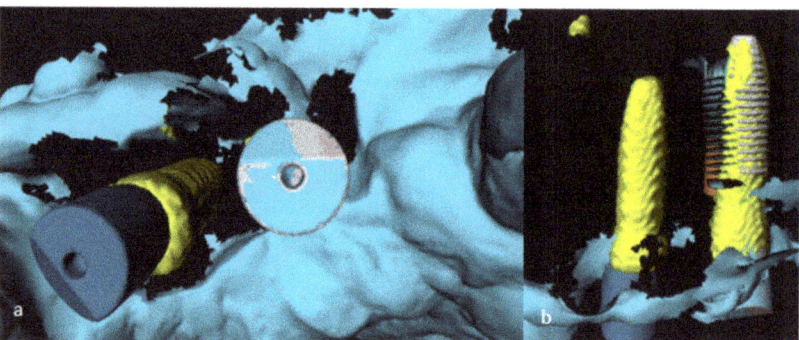

Figure 9. Occlusal (**a**) and subcrestal (**b**) view of two implants.

The sample size of this study is, with a total of 23 implants in 16 participants, relatively small.

For CBCT imaging, a voxel size between 0.25 mm and 0.4 mm was used. The voxel size could influence linear measurements; however, the literature has stated that these differences are not found to be statistical significant [14,15].

VBR and SBR procedures were almost entirely automated, with only the initial alignment of the images carried out manually. The studies of Nada et al. [4] and Baan et al. [16] also compared interobserver variabilities in SBR and showed no significant differences, meaning that matching procedures are highly reproducible.

Regarding the accuracy of both matching procedures, the literature states that VBR displays less variability than SBR. However, differences between both methods were found to be non-significant [5,17]. This indicates that determinations in 3D models by means of SBR and in scans by means of VBR can be compared with each other.

Additionally, a visual check of the VBR between segmented implant and implant model showed an accurate match in most cases. However, in two cases, there was a clear deviation visible between the two tips. These tip deviations obviously influence accuracy results. Shoulders and angulations showed no clear deviations in all cases.

Regarding the accuracy of the IOS and, in particular, the Trios® 3, Pattamavilai and Ongthiemsak [18] and Amornvit et al. [19] showed that this scanner produces an accurate and true representation of the real-life intraoral situation.

In an in vitro setting, Zhou et al. [20] claimed that no significant differences were found between implant location determinations by CBCT or IOS. However, this study compared deviations between postoperative imaging, whereas our study compared deviations between preoperative planning and postoperative implant locations. Furthermore, Zhou et al. [20] matched 3D imaging by manually marking fiducial points. Incorporating manual steps into the matching process allows observational errors. In contrast, in our study, matching and all calculations were automatically conducted. Within the IPOP method, the only manual step is to mark six points on the dental arch, which have been proven to have no significant influence on the accuracy of implant placements [9].

Franchina et al. [21] also compared IOS to CBCT for implant placement accuracy determination in an in vitro setting. This study corroborated that IOS is an alternative relative to CBCT to determine implant placement accuracy.

To our knowledge, only the study of Skjerven et al. [22] compared IOS to CBCT as a method for implant placement accuracy in vivo. They also validated IOS as an alternative to CBCT to determine implant placement accuracies. However, they only measured absolute deviations between implant planning and placement. Again, if the deviations are not corrected for the direction of the deviation, including bucco-lingual and mesio-distal directions, the outcome has hardly any clinical significance.

Furthermore, at least two in vivo studies [23,24] already determined implant placement accuracies by postoperative IOS. However, one of these studies by Derksen et al. [23] stated that additional studies to compare both accuracy evaluation methods are necessary to confirm that a postoperative IOS is a valid alternative to a postoperative CBCT for determining implant placement accuracy.

Future developments in software design will introduce fully automated accuracy-determination processes, enabling the surgeon to determine the accuracy of implant placement preoperatively.

Future studies could focus on using IOS as a method to evaluate implant placement accuracy in fully edentulous patients. Since the IOS does not have any teeth as reference points in these cases, one would think that IOS is not suited for fully edentulous patients.

Additionally, a study with the same design as this study could be carried out again but on a larger group of patients. A power analysis before conducting the study could indicate how many patients are needed and adds more power to the study's findings.

Besides using IOS to assess implant placement accuracies, other non-invasive methods could be further researched in a controlled clinical trial and be compared to CBCT and IOS to determine the accuracy of each of these methods.

5. Conclusions

Our results show that a postoperative IOS is a validated alternative to a postoperative CBCT scan for determining implant placement accuracy.

There were no significant deviations found between CBCT and IOS on the MD-plane and only relatively small, significant deviations on the BL/BP-plane. However, since there are but a few clinical studies comparing IOS to CBCT for the evaluation of implant placement accuracy, additional research is needed to support our statements.

Author Contributions: Conceptualization, F.B., G.M., L.V. and G.K.; methodology, F.B. and J.v.H.; software, F.B., L.V., G.K. and J.v.H.; validation, J.v.H., G.K., E.B. and J.D.; formal analysis, J.v.H., G.K., E.B. and J.D.; investigation, G.K., J.v.H. and G.M.; resources, J.L.; data curation, G.K.; writing—original draft preparation, G.K.; writing—review and editing, J.v.H., J.L., F.B., L.V., G.M. and J.D.; supervision, J.v.H.; project administration, J.v.H. All authors have read and agreed to the published version of the manuscript.

Funding: This research received no external funding.

Institutional Review Board Statement: The study was conducted in accordance with the Declaration of Helsinki and approved by the Ethics Committee of Oost-Nederland (protocol code 2020-6449, 7 May 2020).

Informed Consent Statement: Informed consent was obtained from all subjects involved in the study. Written informed consent has been obtained from patients to publish this paper.

Data Availability Statement: The data presented in this study will be made openly available in DANS EASY data repository after the publication of this manuscript.

Conflicts of Interest: The authors declare no conflict of interest.

References

1. D'Haese, J.; Ackhurst, J.; Wismeijer, D.; De Bruyn, H.; Tahmaseb, A. Current state of the art of computer-guided implant surgery. *Periodontology 2000* **2017**, *73*, 121–133. [CrossRef] [PubMed]
2. Jorba-García, A.; González-Barnadas, A.; Camps-Font, O.; Figueiredo, R.; Valmaseda-Castellón, E. Accuracy assessment of dynamic computer–aided implant placement: A systematic review and meta-analysis. *Clin. Oral Investig.* **2021**, *25*, 2479–2494. [CrossRef] [PubMed]
3. Smitkarn, P.; Subbalekha, K.; Mattheos, N.; Pimkhaokham, A. The accuracy of single-tooth implants placed using fully digital-guided surgery and freehand implant surgery. *J. Clin. Periodontol.* **2019**, *46*, 949–957. [CrossRef] [PubMed]
4. Nada, R.M.; Maal, T.J.J.; Breuning, K.H.; Bergé, S.J.; Mostafa, Y.A.; Kuijpers-Jagtman, A.M. Accuracy and Reproducibility of Voxel Based Superimposition of Cone Beam Computed Tomography Models on the Anterior Cranial Base and the Zygomatic Arches. *PLoS ONE* **2011**, *6*, e16520. [CrossRef] [PubMed]
5. Almukhtar, A.; Ju, X.; Khambay, B.; McDonald, J.; Ayoub, A. Comparison of the Accuracy of Voxel Based Registration and Surface Based Registration for 3D Assessment of Surgical Change following Orthognathic Surgery. *PLoS ONE* **2014**, *9*, e93402. [CrossRef] [PubMed]
6. Jacobs, R.; Salmon, B.; Codari, M.; Hassan, B.; Bornstein, M.M. Cone beam computed tomography in implant dentistry: Recommendations for clinical use. *BMC Oral Health* **2018**, *18*, 88. [CrossRef]
7. Ortorp, A.; Jemt, T.; Bäck, T. Photogrammetry and Conventional Impressions for Recording Implant Positions: A Comparative Laboratory Study. *Clin. Implant Dent. Relat. Res.* **2005**, *7*, 43–50. [CrossRef]
8. Maes, F.; Collignon, A.; Vandermeulen, D.; Marchal, G.; Suetens, P. Multimodality image registration by maximization of mutual information. *IEEE Trans. Med. Imaging* **1997**, *16*, 187–198. [CrossRef]
9. Verhamme, L.M.; Meijer, G.J.; Boumans, T.; Schutyser, F.; Bergé, S.J.; Maal, T.J.J. A clinically relevant validation method for implant placement after virtual planning. *Clin. Oral Implant. Res.* **2013**, *24*, 1265–1272. [CrossRef]
10. Chen, Y.-W.; Hanak, B.W.; Yang, T.-C.; Wilson, T.A.; Hsia, J.M.; Walsh, H.E.; Shih, H.-C.; Nagatomo, K.J. Computer-Assisted Surgery in Medical and Dental Applications. *Expert Rev. Med. Devices* **2021**, *18*, 669–696. [CrossRef]
11. Pellegrino, G.; Taraschi, V.; Andrea, Z.; Ferri, A.; Marchetti, C. Dynamic navigation: A prospective clinical trial to evaluate the accuracy of implant placement. *Int. J. Comput. Dent.* **2019**, *22*, 139–147. [PubMed]
12. Stefanelli, L.V.; DeGroot, B.S.; I Lipton, D.; A Mandelaris, G. Accuracy of a Dynamic Dental Implant Navigation System in a Private Practice. *Int. J. Oral Maxillofac. Implant.* **2019**, *34*, 205–213. [CrossRef] [PubMed]
13. Wu, D.; Zhou, L.; Yang, J.; Zhang, B.; Lin, Y.; Chen, J.; Huang, W.; Chen, Y. Accuracy of dynamic navigation compared to static surgical guide for dental implant placement. *Int. J. Implant Dent.* **2020**, *6*, 78. [CrossRef]
14. Sherrard, J.F.; Rossouw, P.E.; Benson, B.W.; Carrillo, R.; Buschang, P.H. Accuracy and reliability of tooth and root lengths measured on cone-beam computed tomographs. *Am. J. Orthod. Dentofac. Orthop.* **2010**, *137*, S100–S108. [CrossRef]
15. Torres, M.G.G.; Campos, P.S.F.; Segundo, N.P.N.; Navarro, M.; Crusoé-Rebello, I. Accuracy of Linear Measurements in Cone Beam Computed Tomography With Different Voxel Sizes. *Implant Dent.* **2012**, *21*, 150–155. [CrossRef] [PubMed]
16. Baan, F.; Sabelis, J.F.; Schreurs, R.; van de Steeg, G.; Xi, T.; van Riet, T.C.T.; Becking, A.G.; Maal, T.J.J. Validation of the OrthoGnathicAnalyser 2.0-3D accuracy assessment tool for bimaxillary surgery and genioplasty. *PLoS ONE* **2021**, *16*, e0246196. [CrossRef] [PubMed]
17. Han, G.; Li, J.; Wang, S.; Wang, L.; Zhou, Y.; Liu, Y. A comparison of voxel- and surface-based cone-beam computed tomography mandibular superimposition in adult orthodontic patients. *J. Int. Med. Res.* **2021**, *49*, 300060520982708. [CrossRef]
18. Pattamavilai, S.; Ongthiemsak, C. Accuracy of intraoral scanners in different complete arch scan patterns. *J. Prosthet. Dent.* **2022**, *in press*. [CrossRef] [PubMed]
19. Amornvit, P.; Rokaya, D.; Sanohkan, S. Comparison of Accuracy of Current Ten Intraoral Scanners. *BioMed Res. Int.* **2021**, *2021*, 2673040. [CrossRef]
20. Zhou, M.; Zhou, H.; Li, S.-Y.; Geng, Y.-M. Dental implant location via surface scanner: A pilot study. *BMC Oral Health* **2020**, *20*, 306. [CrossRef]
21. Franchina, A.; Stefanelli, L.V.; Maltese, F.; Mandelaris, G.A.; Vantaggiato, A.; Pagliarulo, M.; Pranno, N.; Brauner, E.; De Angelis, F.; Di Carlo, S. Validation of an Intra-Oral Scan Method Versus Cone Beam Computed Tomography Superimposition to Assess

the Accuracy between Planned and Achieved Dental Implants: A Randomized In Vitro Study. *Int. J. Environ. Res. Public Health* **2020**, *17*, 9358. [CrossRef] [PubMed]
22. Skjerven, H.; Olsen-Bergem, H.; Rønold, H.J.; Riis, U.H.; Ellingsen, J.E. Comparison of postoperative intraoral scan versus cone beam computerised tomography to measure accuracy of guided implant placement—A prospective clinical study. *Clin. Oral Implants Res.* **2019**, *30*, 531–541. [CrossRef] [PubMed]
23. Derksen, W.; Wismeijer, D.; Flügge, T.; Hassan, B.; Tahmaseb, A. The accuracy of computer-guided implant surgery with tooth-supported, digitally designed drill guides based on CBCT and intraoral scanning. A prospective cohort study. *Clin. Oral Implants Res.* **2019**, *30*, 1005–1015. [CrossRef] [PubMed]
24. Orban, K.; Varga, E.; Windisch, P.; Braunitzer, G.; Molnar, B. Accuracy of half-guided implant placement with machine-driven or manual insertion: A prospective, randomized clinical study. *Clin. Oral Investig.* **2022**, *26*, 1035–1043. [CrossRef] [PubMed]

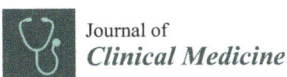

Article

Effect of Scanned Area and Operator on the Accuracy of Dentate Arch Scans with a Single Implant

Vinicius Rizzo Marques [1], Gülce Çakmak [1], Hakan Yilmaz [2], Samir Abou-Ayash [1], Mustafa Borga Donmez [1,3,*] and Burak Yilmaz [1,4,5]

1. Department of Reconstructive Dentistry and Gerodontology, School of Dental Medicine, University of Bern, 3012 Bern, Switzerland; vinicius.rizzo-marques@zmk.unibe.ch (V.R.M.); guelce.cakmak@unibe.ch (G.Ç.); samir.abou-ayash@unibe.ch (S.A.-A.); burak.yilmaz@unibe.ch (B.Y.)
2. İkon Oral and Dental Health Center, Istanbul 34275, Turkey; hakanyilmaz90@gmail.com
3. Department of Prosthodontics, Faculty of Dentistry, Istinye University, Istanbul 34010, Turkey
4. Department of Restorative, Preventive, and Pediatric Dentistry, School of Dental Medicine, University of Bern, 3012 Bern, Switzerland
5. Division of Restorative and Prosthetic Dentistry, The Ohio State University, Columbus, OH 43210, USA
* Correspondence: mustafa-borga.doenmez@unibe.ch

Abstract: Studies have shown the effect of the operator and scanned areas on the accuracy of single implant scans. However, the knowledge on the scan accuracy of the remaining dental arch during single implant scans, which may affect the occlusion, is limited. The aim of this study was to investigate the effect of scanned areas and the operator on the scan accuracy of a dentate arch while scanning a single implant. A dentate model with an anterior implant was digitized with a laboratory scanner (reference scan). Three operators with similar experience performed 10 complete- and 10 partial-arch scans (left 2nd molar to right canine) with an intraoral scanner (TRIOS 3), and these scans were superimposed over the reference. The accuracy was analyzed at 22 points in complete-arch and at 16 points in partial-arch scans on 2nd molars and incisors. Data were evaluated with 2-way ANOVA and Tukey HSD tests ($\alpha = 0.05$). The trueness of the total scanned area was higher in partial- than in complete-arch scans ($p < 0.001$). The trueness and precision of the scans were higher in the anterior site compared with the posterior in complete- (trueness: $p \leq 0.022$, precision: $p \leq 0.003$) and partial-arch (trueness: $p \leq 0.016$, precision: $p \leq 0.016$) scans of each operator and when the operator scan data were pooled. The complete-arch scan's precision was not influenced by the operator ($p \geq 0.029$), whereas the partial-arch scans of operator 1 and 2 were significantly different ($p = 0.036$). Trueness was higher in partial- compared with complete-arch scans, but their precision was similar. Accuracy was higher in the anterior site regardless of the scan being a partial- or a complete-arch. The operator's effect on the accuracy of partial- and complete-arch scans was small.

Keywords: implant scan; operator; precision; scan area; trueness

1. Introduction

The launch of new intraoral scanners (IOSs) and improved accuracy with scanner technologies enabled the fabrication of implant-supported monolithic crowns through a direct digital workflow with clinically acceptable accuracy and less patient discomfort in recent years [1–7]. However, studies focusing on varying clinical scenarios are still conducted to identify the factors affecting the scan accuracy [7–11] such as scanned area and operator experience [11–19]. Regarding the effect of operator experience on scan accuracy, conflicting results have been reported [18,20,21]. Operator experience did not affect the accuracy in some studies. Contrarily, in others, operator experience did affect the accuracy [18,19,22,23]. The operators had different levels of experience, and different study protocols were applied in those studies. Clinicians may have similar experience in scanning. However, it is not well known if the accuracy of their scans would still be similar.

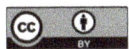

Therefore, it is essential to further investigate the various factors that affect the accurate transfer of the position of the implant, its relation with the remainder of the arch, and the scan accuracy of the entire arch, not just the implant's itself.

Teeth act as fixed reference points and facilitate image acquisition and stitching during image acquisition [24]. Therefore, intraoral scans of a dentate arch have been reported to have acceptable accuracy [8,24]. However, conflicting results were reported for the accuracy of the scans when the scans were restricted to anterior or posterior regions of a dentate arch [25,26]. This could be attributed to the geometry difference in anterior and posterior teeth, which is known to affect the proper alignment [24,26], curvature of the arch [19,20,25,27] and the extent of the scanned area [23,25]. In a previous study, the accuracy tended to decrease from anterior to posterior teeth in the scans of a dentate arch [26]. Additionally, depending on the scanned region, complete- or partial-arch scans differed in accuracy of a dentate arch [28].

For single implant or prepared natural tooth scans, clinically acceptable accuracy was attributed to the limited extent of the scanned area when the arch was scanned partially [29–31]. Although complete-arch scans have the possibility of incurring misalignment errors with the increased scanned area and number of stitched images [17,20,22], complete-arch scans are still commonly performed for single implant scans [32]. Studies have shown that partial-arch scans can be as accurate as complete-arch scans, and recommended the use of partial-arch scans for implants both in the anterior and posterior regions [1,25,33,34]. However, those studies [1,25] focused on the accuracy of only the implant position. The scan accuracy of the remainder of the arch can also be crucial even though it may not directly affect the accuracy or the fit of an implant-supported crown. Clinicians primarily focus on the implant site during scanning, which may affect the accuracy of the rest of the arch. Dental arch accuracy may affect occlusion if deviations from the intraoral situation exist [25,33]. In addition, depending on the deviation's magnitude and location, scan accuracy of the dental arch may affect the definitive restoration [33,35]. Therefore, the present study aimed to compare the trueness and precision of dental arches in scans during digitization of a single implant either with partial- or complete-arch scans. The accuracy of anterior and posterior sites was also aimed to be compared within and between the partial- and complete-arch scans when three different operators performed the scans. The null hypotheses were the following: (1) the scanned area (partial- vs. complete-arch) and the operator would not affect the accuracy of scans of the total scanned area; (2) the scan accuracy of the site (anterior vs. posterior left vs. posterior right in complete-arch and anterior vs. posterior left in partial-arch) would not be different for pooled data from all operators and for each operator, within each scan group; and (3) the accuracy of anterior sites and posterior sites would not be affected by the scan being complete- or partial-arch and the operator being also tested.

2. Materials and Methods

2.1. Data Acquisition

A partially edentulous maxillary model with an implant (4.0 × 11 mm) (Proactive Straight Implant; Neoss, Woodland Hills, CA, USA), and an intraoral scan body (Intra-Oral Scanbody, Neoss, Woodland Hills, CA, USA) at left central incisor site was additively manufactured (Form 2, Formlabs Inc., Somerville, MA, USA) [1]. A laboratory scanner with 4 μm accuracy was used (Ceramill Map 600, Amann Girrbach AG, Koblach, Austria) to obtain a reference scan of the model. Ten complete-arch scans (Figure 1) were performed with an IOS with 6.9 μm accuracy (TRIOS 3 v 1.4.7.5, 3Shape, Copenhagen, Denmark) by 3 operators with similar scanning experience (2 years of experience with intraoral scanning and at least 10 pilot scans with the IOS used). Partial-arch scans (Figure 2) were also performed by the same operators, from the distal of left 2nd molar to the distal of right canine (n = 10). The scan order was randomized by using a software program (Excel, Microsoft Corp, Redmond, WA, USA). A scan path, which was recommended by the manufacturer of the scanner, was followed for all scans, from the occlusal of left 2nd molars, continuing onto the occlusals/incisals of remaining teeth in each group followed by their lingual and buccal surfaces. All scans were performed in the same temperature-(20 °C) and humidity-controlled (45%) room, which was lit by sunlight and had an air pressure of 750 ± 5 mm [36].

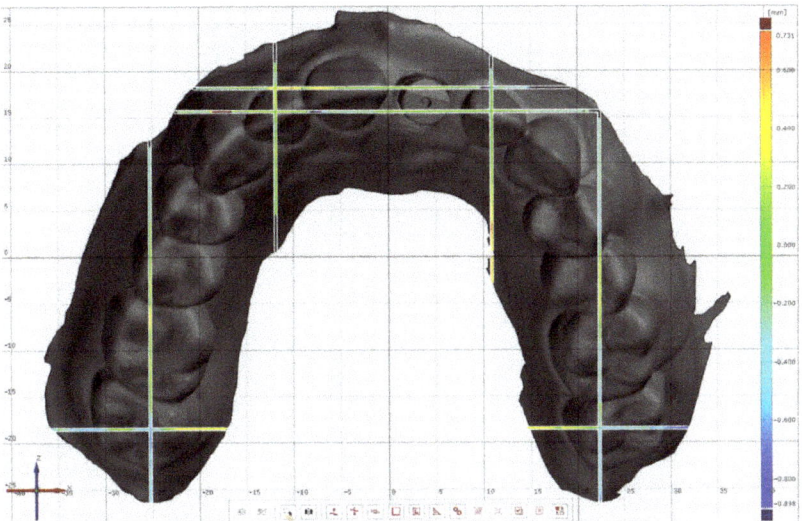

Figure 1. Complete-arch intraoral scan including the planes for subsequent analyses.

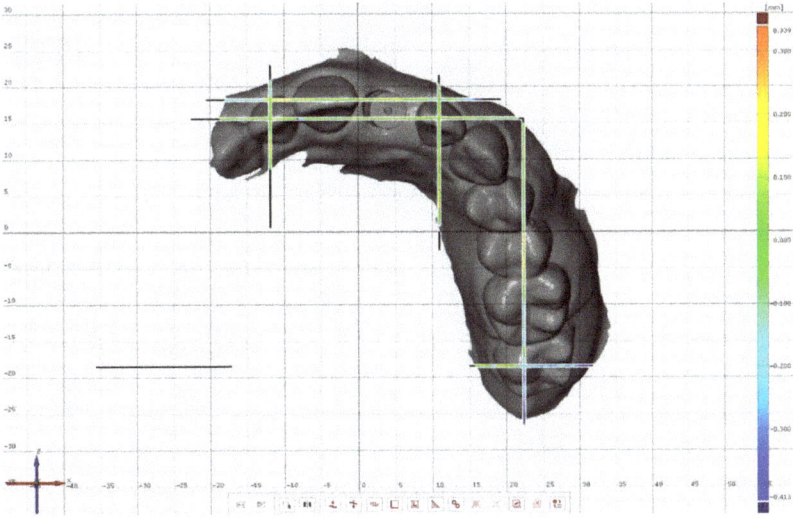

Figure 2. Partial-arch intraoral scan, including the planes for subsequent analyses.

2.2. Evaluation of Accuracy

The IOS's scans were converted to standard tessellation (STL) files and exported to a 3-dimensional metrology software (Pro 8.1, GOM GmbH, Braunschweig, Germany) for comparisons with the reference scan. For the superimposition of reference and complete-arch scanned models, initially the GOM's software prealignment feature was used, and all teeth and the scan body were selected for further alignment by using the "local best-fit" tool. On partial-arch scans, the area for superimpositions selected was from the distal of left 2nd molar to the distal of right lateral incisor. For evaluation, 4 planes in buccopalatal orientation were generated on the reference scan that passed through the distopalatal cusp of the 2nd molars and at the center of lateral incisors; and 3 planes in the mesiodistal orientation that passed through the center of the occlusal surface of 2nd molars, mesial of lateral incisors, and mesial of right central incisor. For complete-arch scans (Figure 3), 22 points were selected on 7 planes on 2nd molars and incisors at the gingival margin and the most incisal point both on buccopalatal and mesiodistal planes. For partial-arch scans (Figure 4), the mesiodistal plane and corresponding points on the right 2nd molar were not evaluated as that region was not captured with the IOS, resulting in 16 points on 6 planes. All coordinates for predefined planes and points were added, and the software algorithm generated the 3-dimensional (3D) variation between the points on the reference and the test scans.

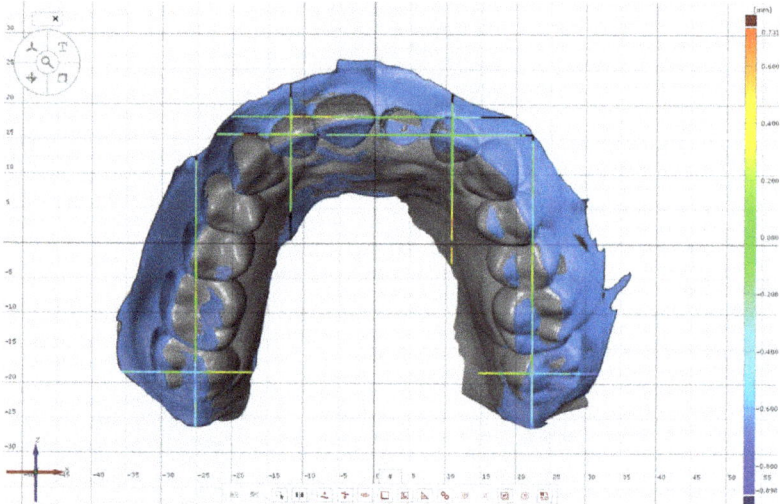

Figure 3. Measurement points (Left 2nd molar: Buccal, palatal, and distal gingival margins, mesiopalatal and distopalatal cusp tips, and most buccal point of the tooth. Left lateral incisor: Buccal, palatal, and mesial gingival margins, most mesial and incisal point of the tooth. Right central incisor: Mesial gingival margin and most mesial point of the tooth. Right lateral incisor: Buccal and gingival margins and most incisal point of the tooth. Right 2nd molar: Buccal, palatal, and distal gingival margins, mesiopalatal and distopalatal cusp tips, and most buccal point of the tooth) on complete-arch scan at selected planes when superimposed to the reference scan.

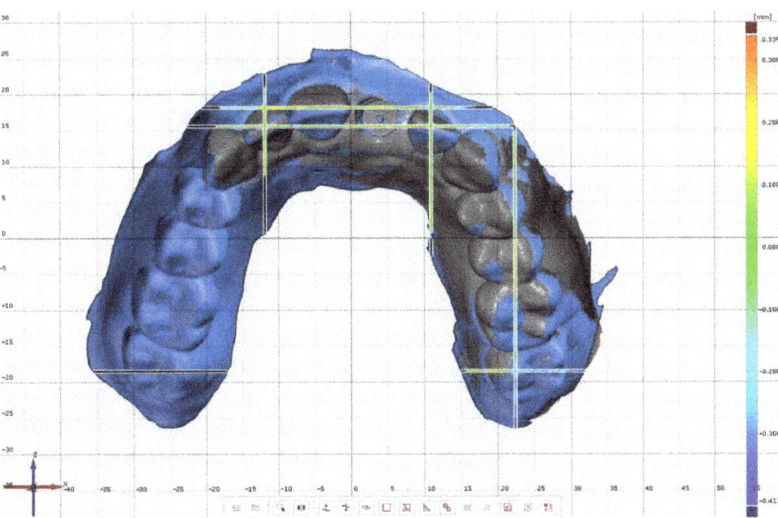

Figure 4. Measurement points (Left 2nd molar: Buccal, palatal, and distal gingival margins, mesiopalatal and distopalatal cusp tips, and most buccal point of the tooth. Left lateral incisor: Buccal, palatal, and mesial gingival margins, most mesial and incisal point of the tooth. Right central incisor: Mesial gingival margin and most mesial point of the tooth. Right lateral incisor: Buccal and gingival margins and most incisal point of the tooth) on partial-arch scan at selected planes when superimposed to the reference scan.

2.3. Statistical Analysis

The data generated (3D distance deviation at all points, Figure 5) were used (Excel, Microsoft Corp, Seattle, WA, USA) for statistical analysis. The homogeneity of variances was analyzed by using Levene's test, and a 2-way analysis of variance (ANOVA) followed by Tukey HSD were used to analyze the effect of the scanned area, the operator, and their interaction on trueness and precision of scans ($\alpha = 0.05$).

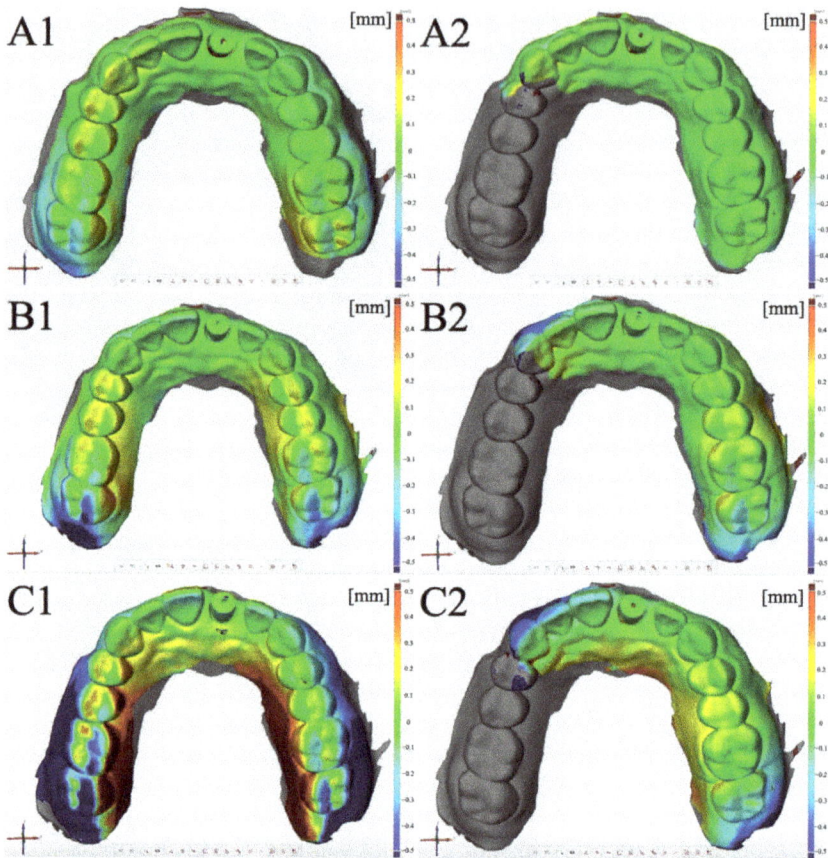

Figure 5. Color maps generated by the superimposition of test scans over reference scan: (**A**) Operator 1. (**B**) Operator 2. (**C**) Operator 3. (**1**) Complete-arch scan. (**2**) Partial-arch scan.

3. Results

When the effect of the operator on the scanned area was considered, the two-way ANOVA revealed that only the scanned area affected the trueness of total area scanned ($p < 0.001$). Partial-arch scans had higher trueness than the complete-arch scans ($p < 0.001$). There was no significant difference among the operators in terms of the trueness of total scanned area in complete- ($p \geq 0.214$) and partial-arch scans ($p \geq 0.073$) (Table 1).

Table 1. Two-way ANOVA results for trueness and precision.

Property	Effect	Df	F-Ratio	p-Value
	Operator	2	2.671	0.070
Trueness (μm)	Scanned area	1	24.706	<0.001
	Operator × Scanned area	2	0.763	0.467
	Operator	2	1.067	0.344
Precision (μm)	Scanned area	1	1.379	0.241
	Operator × Scanned area	2	4.505	0.011

df, numerator degrees of freedom.

When the trueness was analyzed within scanned areas (complete- or partial-arch) (Table 2), for complete-arch scans, anterior sites had higher trueness than left posterior sites, which had higher trueness than right posterior sites overall (pooled data from all operators) ($p < 0.001$) and for each operators' scans (for operator 1: $p \leq 0.022$, for operator 2 and 3: $p < 0.001$) (Figure 6). For partial-arch scans, the anterior site had higher trueness than the left posterior site, overall (pooled data from all operators) ($p < 0.001$) and for all operators ($p < 0.001$ for operators 1 and 3, $p = 0.016$ for operator 2).

Table 2. Mean and standard deviation values for trueness and precision of complete and partial arch scans from different operators and pooled data from all operators.

Parameter	Arch	Area	Operator 1	Operator 2	Operator 3	Operator Pooled
Trueness (μm)	Complete	Ant	273.2 ± 544.9 [A,1]	217.9 ± 404.3 [A,1]	243.9 ± 420.8 [A,1]	245.3 ± 462.0 [A,1]
		Left Post	568.2 ± 735.2 [B,2]	672.3 ± 767.9 [B,2]	710.3 ± 831.6 [B,2]	648.2 ± 774.3 [B,2]
		Right Post	1088.4 ± 667.4 [C]	1196.4 ± 596.6 [C]	1354.7 ± 604.9 [C]	1208.3 ± 630.2 [C]
		Total	583.7 ± 717.87 *	621.0 ± 704.4 *	686.3 ± 760.0 *	628.3 ± 726.6
	Partial	Ant	178.9 ± 287.5 [D,1]	374.2 ± 676.1 [D,1]	285.4 ± 457.7 [D,1]	286.1 ± 515.6 [D,1]
		Left Post	544.5 ± 740.8 [E,2]	673.0 ± 766.7 [E,2]	739.8 ± 827.2 [E,2]	656.1 ± 779.1 [E,2]
		Total	310.5 ± 527.6 *	475.2 ± 719.5 *	443.2 ± 646.4 *	414.8 ± 643.7
Precision (μm)	Complete	Ant	350.1 ± 415.7 [A,1]	253.4 ± 311.7 [A,1]	254.2 ± 332.2 [A,1]	287.3 ± 358.9 [A,1]
		Left Post	579.6 ± 444.3 [B,3]	596.1 ± 476.2 [B,3]	650.2 ± 509.0 [B,2]	607.2 ± 473.7 [B,2]
		Right Post	575.4 ± 330.6 [B]	519.5 ± 286.0 [B]	531.3 ± 279.6 [B]	542.4 ± 299.5 [B]
		Total	472.0 ± 414.2 *	416.5 ± 382.8 *	432.4 ± 406.0 *	440.6 ± 401.1
	Partial	Ant	217.1 ± 186.7 [C,2]	374.7 ± 676.2 [C,2]	303.5 ± 340.8 [C,1]	334.8 ± 383.8 [C,1]
		Left Post	485.8 ± 666.6 [D,3]	673.2 ± 766.9 [D,3]	654.1 ± 496.8 [D,2]	612.6 ± 478.6 [D,2]
		Total	313.8 ± 443.4 *	475.5 ± 719.6 †	425.2 ± 433.8 *,†	409.7 ± 557.3

Ant, anterior; post, posterior. Significant differences among scanned sites are presented by using different uppercase superscript letters in the same column for complete- and partial-arch, independently. Significant differences between the same scanned sites (anterior or left posterior) of partial- and complete-arch scans are presented by using different numbers in the same column. Significant differences between total trueness and precision of operator groups of complete- and partial-arch scans are presented by using different symbols in the same row.

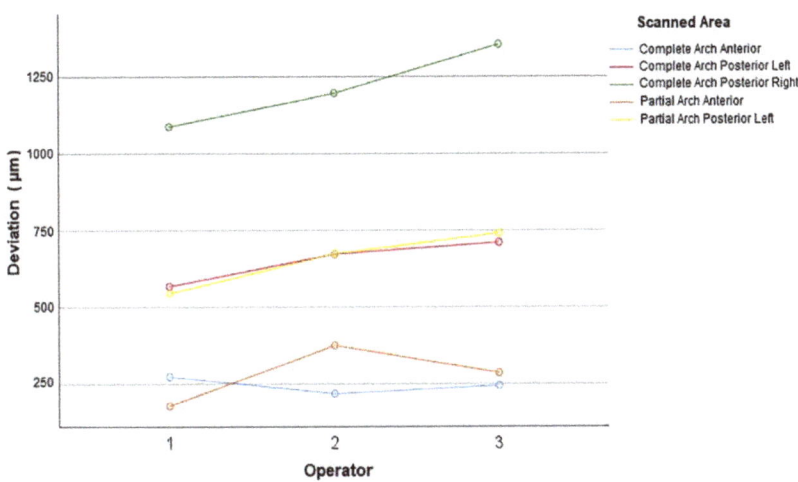

Figure 6. Deviations (indicating trueness) of different sites in complete- and partial-arch scans for each operator.

When the effect of the scanned area on trueness at anterior sites was considered by analyzing the pooled data from all operators ($p = 0.33$) and for each operator ($p \geq 0.056$), no significant difference was found between partial- and complete-arch scans.

When the effect of the scanned area on trueness at left posterior sites was considered by analyzing the pooled data from all operators ($p = 0.93$) and for each operator ($p \geq 0.863$), no significant difference was found between partial- and complete-arch scans.

For the precision of the total area scanned, the interaction between the operator and the scanned area was significant ($p = 0.011$). There was no significant difference among the operators in terms of total precision in complete-arch scans ($p \geq 0.294$), whereas partial-arch scans of operator 1 had higher precision than the partial-arch scans of operator 2 ($p = 0.036$). No significant difference was observed in other operator pairs of partial-arch scans ($p \geq 0.207$).

When the precision of complete-arch scans was considered by analyzing the pooled data from all operators, precision at anterior sites was higher than that at right and left posterior sites ($p < 0.001$), and no difference was found in precision for left and right posterior sites ($p = 0.367$). The same result was obtained when each operators' scans were individually analyzed ($p \leq 0.003$ for anterior vs. posteriors, $p = 0.998$ for operator 1, $p = 0.494$ for operator 2, and $p = 0.252$ for operator 3 for left to right comparison) (Figure 7).

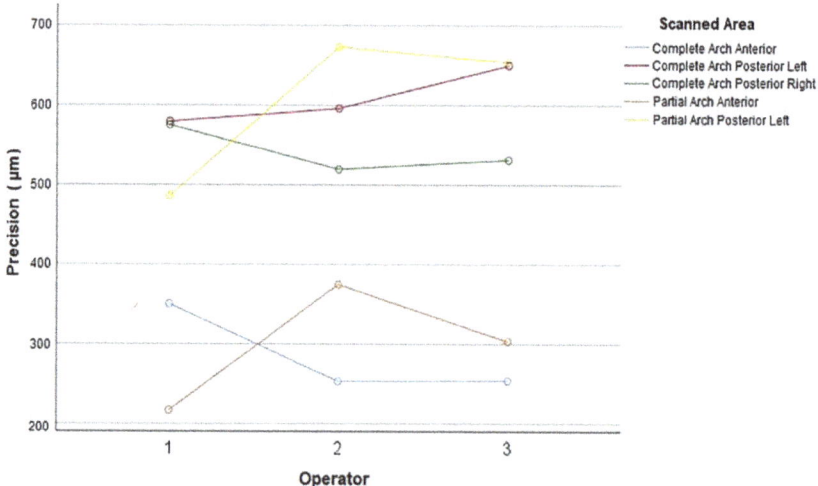

Figure 7. Precision of scans at different sites in complete- and partial-arch scans for each operator.

When the precision of partial-arch scans was considered by analyzing the pooled data from all operators, the precision at anterior sites was higher than the precision at left posterior sites ($p < 0.001$). The precision was higher at the anterior site when the data were analyzed for each operator ($p \leq 0.001$ for operator 1 and 3, and $p = 0.016$ for operator 2).

When the effect of the scanned area on the precision at anterior sites was considered by analyzing the pooled data from all operators ($p = 0.124$) and operator 3 ($p = 0.334$), no significant difference was found between partial- and complete-arch scans. For operator 1, the precision of anterior sites was higher in partial-arch scans than that at complete-arch scans ($p = 0.008$), whereas for operator 2, the precision of anterior sites was lower in partial-arch scans than that in complete-arch scans ($p = 0.001$).

When the effect of the scanned area on the precision at left posterior sites was considered by analyzing the pooled data from all operators, no significant difference was found between partial- and complete-arch scans ($p = 0.974$). The precision at left posterior sites was not significantly different between complete- and partial-arch scans when analyzed for each operator ($p \geq 0.906$).

4. Discussion

The scanned area affected the trueness, and an interaction was found between the operator and the scanned area in terms of precision. Therefore, the first null hypothesis that the scanned area and the operator would not affect the accuracy of total scanned area was rejected. Scan accuracy in the anterior site was higher than that in the posterior site for both the complete- and partial-arch scans of all operators and their pooled data. Therefore, the 2nd null hypothesis was rejected. The operator and the scanned area affected the precision of the scans. Therefore, the 3rd null hypothesis that the accuracy of anterior and posterior sites would not be affected by the scan being complete-arch or partial-arch was rejected.

Direct comparison of the present study results with previous studies is difficult because previous studies focused on the accuracy of single implants (i.e., the scan bodies) [1,5] rather than the accuracy of scans of adjacent teeth and the arch. However, the positional accuracy of the arch is as important as that of the scan body for clinical success of implant-supported restorations. An inaccurately scanned arch may affect the 3D position of the restoration and its interproximal and occlusal contacts and contour [33,35]. Although the fit of the restoration may be acceptable, the restoration may need proximal and/or occlusal contact adjustments, including trimming or additional ceramic application, further glazing and/or polishing steps [33,35]. An over- or under-countoured restoration may affect the esthetics and hygiene, and thus require adjustments. When the restoration is made in monolithic form out of a CAD-CAM material and is under-contoured, additional ceramic or composite resin application on occlusal or proximal contacts may be problematic. Chipping can be a further clinical problem when ceramic or composite resin is applied over monolithic CAD-CAM ceramics or composite resins, since monolithic restorations are designed without cutback. The inaccuracy in the proximal contacts may affect the insertion axis of the crown, the path of withdrawal, and its proper seating. These additional adjustment steps may increase the time spent chairside and may decrease the efficacy of the direct digital workflow and comfort of the clinician and the patient. In addition, with screw-retained restorations, the location of the access hole within the overall crown shape may be improper, as the outer crown contours may deviate from the ideal. The above-mentioned issues may be encountered considering the high deviation values in the posterior region in the present study, and the deviation values exceed 1 mm in some areas.

Previously, the scans of incisal surfaces of the anterior teeth were reported to be difficult and more prone to errors during the alignment because of their simple geometries, whereas posterior teeth were reported easier to scan and align because of the complex geometries of occlusal surfaces on molars and premolars [24]. However, in the present study, higher accuracy was obtained in the anterior site than in the posterior in complete- and partial-arch scans. The presence of the scan body, which has a wider upper surface area compared to the incisal surfaces of the incisors, might have helped for the proper alignment of scans in the anterior site and decreased the deviation. Another contributing factor for increased accuracy in the anterior region may be the linear scanning path of the arch in the anterior region [27]. The scans of the implant used in the present study, which was located in the anterior region, has been reported to be acceptable.

In complete-arch scans, left posterior sites had higher trueness than the right posterior sites, whereas their precision was similar. In the present study, the scans started from the left side of the model. Therefore, lower trueness with the right side may be attributed to the increased number of stitched images and the possibility of increased inherent errors and misalignment of errors when the scanned area increased [23]. Low accuracy was reported in previous studies in the extended scanned areas [23,25,28].

In the present study, trueness at anterior and left posterior sites and the precision at left posterior sites was similar between complete- and partial-arch scans independent of operator. However, while the partial-arch scans of operator 1 had higher precision than that of complete-arch scans at the anterior site, the exact opposite was observed for operator 2. Given that operator 1 also had higher scan precision than operator 2 when partial-arch scans were considered, this result seems consistent. Even though the operators in the present study had similar experience, more reliable results can be obtained and any significant differences among operators may be elaborated thoroughly with the involvement of more operators. Nevertheless, many previous studies used three operators to investigate the effect of the operator on scan accuracy [21,23,37].

The present study was performed under standardized laboratory conditions without including patient specific factors, and the intraoral conditions and results may differ if patient-specific factors are involved [17,35]. In addition, considering that scan accuracy of IOSs is also affected by environmental conditions [1], other in vitro studies might have different results. Previous studies reported that IOS technology and scan path might affect the accuracy of implant scans [17,20], thus the findings may vary depending on the scanner technology and scan path. The use of a laboratory scanner to obtain the reference scans is a limitation. However, the accuracy of the applied laboratory scanner is high, and the application of laboratory scanners to obtain reference datasets has been recommended [38–41]. Future studies should be performed by using an industrial grade scanner for high-accuracy reference scans. The present study results should be validated further by fabricating definitive single unit implant crowns and evaluating their relationship with adjacent teeth and antagonists. Future clinical studies are necessary to corroborate the findings of the present in vitro study.

5. Conclusions

The accuracy of intraoral scans obtained with the IOS used was significantly affected by the scans being partial- or complete-arch. Partial-arch scans had higher trueness than the complete-arch scans, but their precision was similar. The accuracy of the total scanned area was similar among different operators' scans. When the accuracy of scans at different sites in the arch is considered, anterior sites had higher accuracy compared to posterior sites for both partial- and complete-arch scans. In terms of the operator's effect on trueness and precision of scans at different sites in the arch, significant differences were only observed in the precision of anterior site scans of two operators. The scan accuracy of the operators was similar for the remainder of the sites evaluated.

Author Contributions: Conceptualization, V.R.M.; Formal analysis, H.Y.; Investigation, V.R.M. and G.Ç.; Methodology, G.Ç.; Supervision, B.Y.; Writing—original draft, V.R.M., S.A.-A. and M.B.D. All authors have read and agreed to the published version of the manuscript.

Funding: This research received no external funding.

Institutional Review Board Statement: Not applicable.

Informed Consent Statement: Not applicable.

Data Availability Statement: Data sharing is not applicable for this paper.

Conflicts of Interest: The authors declare no conflict of interest.

References

1. Yilmaz, B.; Rizzo, M.V.; Guo, X.; Gouveia, D.; Abou-Ayash, S. The effect of scanned area on the accuracy and time of anterior single implant scans: An in vitro study. *J. Dent.* **2021**, *109*, 103620. [CrossRef] [PubMed]
2. Joda, T.; Brägger, U. Complete digital workflow for the production of implant-supported single-unit monolithic crowns. *Clin. Oral Implants Res.* **2014**, *25*, 1304–1306. [CrossRef]
3. Joda, T.; Ferrari, M.; Gallucci, G.O.; Wittneben, J.G.; Brägger, U. Digital technology in fixed implant prosthodontics. *Periodontology 2000* **2017**, *73*, 178–192. [CrossRef] [PubMed]
4. Michelinakis, G.; Apostolakis, D.; Kamposiora, P.; Papavasiliou, G.; Özcan, M. The direct digital workflow in fixed implant prosthodontics: A narrative review. *BMC Oral Health* **2021**, *21*, 37. [CrossRef] [PubMed]
5. Mühlemann, S.; Greter, E.A.; Park, J.M.; Hämmerle, C.H.F.; Thoma, D.S. Precision of digital implant models compared to conventional implant models for posterior single implant crowns: A within-subject comparison. *Clin. Oral Implants Res.* **2018**, *29*, 931–936. [CrossRef] [PubMed]
6. Lo Giudice, R.; Famà, F. Health care and health service digital revolution. *Int. J. Environ. Res. Public Health* **2020**, *17*, 4913. [CrossRef]

7. De Oliveira, N.R.C.; Pigozzo, M.N.; Sesma, N.; Laganá, D.C. Clinical efficiency and patient preference of digital and conventional workflow for single implant crowns using immediate and regular digital impression: A meta-analysis. *Clin. Oral Implants Res.* **2020**, *31*, 669–686. [CrossRef]
8. Haddadi, Y.; Bahrami, G.; Isidor, F. Accuracy of crowns based on digital intraoral scanning compared to conventional impression-a split-mouth randomised clinical study. *Clin. Oral Investig.* **2019**, *23*, 4043–4050. [CrossRef]
9. Kihara, H.; Hatakeyama, W.; Komine, F.; Takafuji, K.; Takahashi, T.; Yokota, J.; Oriso, K.; Kondo, H. Accuracy and practicality of intraoral scanner in dentistry: A literature review. *J. Prosthodont. Res.* **2020**, *64*, 109–113. [CrossRef]
10. Takeuchi, Y.; Koizumi, H.; Furuchi, M.; Sato, Y.; Ohkubo, C.; Matsumura, H. Use of digital impression systems with intraoral scanners for fabricating restorations and fixed dental prostheses. *J. Oral. Sci.* **2018**, *60*, 1–7. [CrossRef]
11. Schimmel, M.; Akino, N.; Srinivasan, M.; Wittneben, J.G.; Yilmaz, B.; Abou-Ayash, S. Accuracy of intraoral scanning in completely and partially edentulous maxillary and mandibular jaws: An in vitro analysis. *Clin. Oral Investig.* **2021**, *25*, 1839–1847. [PubMed]
12. Rutkūnas, V.; Gečiauskaitė, A.; Jegelevičius, D.; Vaitiekūnas, M. Accuracy of digital implant impressions with intraoral scanners. A systematic review. *Eur. J. Oral Implantol.* **2017**, *10* (Suppl. S1), 101–120. [PubMed]
13. Revilla-León, M.; Jiang, P.; Sadeghpour, M.; Piedra-Cascón, W.; Zandinejad, A.; Özcan, M.; Krishnamurthy, V.R. Intraoral digital scans-Part 1: Influence of ambient scanning light conditions on the accuracy (trueness and precision) of different intraoral scanners. *J. Prosthet. Dent.* **2020**, *124*, 372–378. [CrossRef]
14. Zimmermann, M.; Ender, A.; Mehl, A. Local accuracy of actual intraoral scanning systems for single-tooth preparations in vitro. *J. Am. Dent. Assoc.* **2020**, *151*, 127–135. [CrossRef] [PubMed]
15. Mizumoto, R.M.; Yilmaz, B. Intraoral scan bodies in implant dentistry: A systematic review. *J. Prosthet. Dent.* **2018**, *120*, 343–352. [PubMed]
16. Kim, J.; Park, J.M.; Kim, M.; Heo, S.J.; Shin, I.H.; Kim, M. Comparison of experience curves between two 3-dimensional intraoral scanners. *J. Prosthet. Dent.* **2016**, *116*, 221–230. [CrossRef] [PubMed]
17. Çakmak, G.; Yilmaz, H.; Treviño, A.; Kökat, A.M.; Yilmaz, B. The effect of scanner type and scan body position on the accuracy of complete-arch digital implant scans. *Clin. Implant Dent. Relat. Res.* **2020**, *22*, 533–541. [CrossRef]
18. Ciocca, L.; Meneghello, R.; Monaco, C.S.G.; Scheda, L.; Gatto, M.R.; Baldissara, P. In vitro assessment of the accuracy of digital impressions prepared using a single system for full-arch restorations on implants. *Int. J. Comput. Assist. Radiol. Surg.* **2018**, *13*, 1097–1108. [CrossRef]
19. Giménez, B.; Özcan, M.; Martínez-Rus, F.; Pradíes, G. Accuracy of a digital impression system based on active wavefront sampling technology for implants considering operator experience, implant angulation, and depth. *Clin. Implant Dent. Relat. Res.* **2015**, *17* (Suppl. S1), e54–e64. [CrossRef]
20. Giménez, B.; Pradíes, G.; Martínez-Rus, F.; Özcan, M. Accuracy of two digital implant impression systems based on confocal microscopy with variations in customized software and clinical parameters. *Int. J. Oral Maxillofac. Implants* **2015**, *30*, 56–64. [CrossRef]
21. Arcuri, L.; Pozzi, A.; Lio, F.; Rompen, E.; Zechner, W.; Nardi, A. Influence of implant scanbody material, position and operator on the accuracy of digital impression for complete-arch: A randomized in vitro trial. *J. Prosthodont. Res.* **2020**, *64*, 128–136. [CrossRef] [PubMed]
22. Gimenez-Gonzalez, B.; Hassan, B.; Özcan, M.; Pradíes, G. An in vitro study of factors influencing the performance of digital intraoral impressions operating on active wavefront sampling technology with multiple implants in the edentulous maxilla. *J. Prosthodont.* **2017**, *26*, 650–655. [CrossRef] [PubMed]
23. Resende, C.C.D.; Barbosa, T.A.Q.; Moura, G.F.; Tavares, L.D.N.; Rizzante, F.A.P.; George, F.M.; Neves, F.D.D.; Mendonça, G. Influence of operator experience, scanner type, and scan size on 3D scans. *J. Prosthet. Dent.* **2021**, *125*, 294–299. [CrossRef] [PubMed]
24. Braian, M.; Wennerberg, A. Trueness and precision of 5 intraoral scanners for scanning edentulous and dentate complete-arch mandibular casts: A comparative in vitro study. *J. Prosthet. Dent.* **2019**, *122*, 129–136.e2. [CrossRef] [PubMed]
25. Ender, A.; Zimmermann, M.; Mehl, A. Accuracy of complete- and partial-arch impressions of actual intraoral scanning systems in vitro. *Int. J. Comput. Dent.* **2019**, *22*, 11–19.
26. Son, K.; Lee, K.B. Effect of tooth types on the accuracy of dental 3d scanners: An in vitro study. *Materials* **2020**, *13*, 1744. [CrossRef]
27. Mizumoto, R.M.; Alp, G.; Özcan, M.; Yilmaz, B. The effect of scanning the palate and scan body position on the accuracy of complete-arch implant scans. *Clin. Implant Dent. Relat. Res.* **2019**, *21*, 987–994. [CrossRef]
28. Moon, Y.G.; Lee, K.M. Comparison of the accuracy of intraoral scans between complete-arch scan and quadrant scan. *Prog. Orthod.* **2020**, *21*, 36. [CrossRef]
29. Henkel, G.L. A comparison of fixed prostheses generated from conventional vs digitally scanned dental impressions. *Compend. Contin. Educ. Dent.* **2007**, *28*, 422–424, 426–428, 430–431.
30. Syrek, A.; Reich, G.; Ranftl, D.; Klein, C.; Cerny, B.; Brodesser, J. Clinical evaluation of all-ceramic crowns fabricated from intraoral digital impressions based on the principle of active wavefront sampling. *J. Dent.* **2010**, *38*, 553–559. [CrossRef]
31. Brawek, P.K.; Wolfart, S.; Endres, L.; Kirsten, A.; Reich, S. The clinical accuracy of single crowns exclusively fabricated by digital workflow–the comparison of two systems. *Clin. Oral Investig.* **2013**, *17*, 2119–2125. [CrossRef]
32. Schepke, U.; Meijer, H.J.; Kerdijk, W.; Cune, M.S. Digital versus analog complete-arch impressions for single-unit premolar implant crowns: Operating time and patient preference. *J. Prosthet. Dent.* **2015**, *114*, 403–406.e1. [CrossRef] [PubMed]
33. Zhang, Y.; Tian, J.; Wei, D.; Di, P.; Lin, Y. Quantitative clinical adjustment analysis of posterior single implant crown in a chairside digital workflow: A randomized controlled trial. *Clin. Oral Implants Res.* **2019**, *30*, 1059–1066. [CrossRef] [PubMed]

34. De Angelis, P.; Passarelli, P.C.; Gasparini, G.; Boniello, R.; D'Amato, G.; De Angelis, S. Monolithic CAD-CAM lithium disilicate versus monolithic CAD-CAM zirconia for single implant-supported posterior crowns using a digital workflow: A 3-year cross-sectional retrospective study. *J. Prosthet. Dent.* **2020**, *123*, 252–256. [CrossRef] [PubMed]
35. Lee, S.J.; Jamjoom, F.Z.; Le, T.; Radics, A.; Gallucci, G.O. A clinical study comparing digital scanning and conventional impression making for implant-supported prostheses: A crossover clinical trial. *J. Prosthet. Dent.* **2021**. *online ahead of print*. [CrossRef]
36. Donmez, M.B.; Çakmak, G.; Atalay, S.; Yilmaz, H.; Yilmaz, B. Trueness and precision of combined healing abutment-scan body system depending on the scan pattern and implant location: An in-vitro study. *J. Dent.* **2022**, 104169. [CrossRef]
37. Revilla-León, M.; Subramanian, S.G.; Özcan, M.; Krishnamurthy, V.R. Clinical study of the influence of ambient light scanning conditions on the accuracy (trueness and precision) of an intraoral scanner. *J. Prosthodont.* **2020**, *29*, 107–113. [CrossRef]
38. Atalay, S.; Çakmak, G.; Donmez, M.B.; Yilmaz, H.; Kökat, A.M.; Yilmaz, B. Effect of implant location and operator on the accuracy of implant scans using a combined healing abutment-scan body system. *J. Dent.* **2021**, *115*, 103855. [CrossRef]
39. You, S.M.; You, S.G.; Kang, S.Y.; Bae, S.Y.; Kim, J.H. Evaluation of the accuracy (trueness and precision) of a maxillary trial denture according to the layer thickness: An in vitro study. *J. Prosthet. Dent.* **2021**, *125*, 139–145. [CrossRef]
40. Kim, J.H.; Son, S.A.; Lee, H.; Kim, R.J.; Park, J.K. In vitro analysis of intraoral digital impression of inlay preparation according to tooth location and cavity type. *J. Prosthodont. Res.* **2021**, *65*, 400–406. [CrossRef]
41. Pan, Y.; Tsoi, J.K.H.; Lam, W.Y.H.; Pow, E.H.N. Implant framework misfit: A systematic review on assessment methods and clinical complications. *Clin. Implant Dent. Relat. Res.* **2021**, *23*, 244–258. [CrossRef] [PubMed]

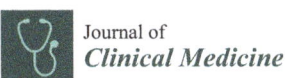

Article

Update on the Accuracy of Conventional and Digital Full-Arch Impressions of Partially Edentulous and Fully Dentate Jaws in Young and Elderly Subjects: A Clinical Trial

Maximiliane Amelie Schlenz *, Julian Maximilian Stillersfeld, Bernd Wöstmann and Alexander Schmidt

Department of Prosthodontics, Dental Clinic, Justus Liebig University, Schlangenzahl 14, 35392 Giessen, Germany; julian.m.stillersfeld@dentist.med.uni-giessen.de (J.M.S.); bernd.woestmann@dentist.med.uni-giessen.de (B.W.); alexander.schmidt@dentist.med.uni-giessen.de (A.S.)
* Correspondence: maximiliane.a.schlenz@dentist.med.uni-giessen.de

Citation: Schlenz, M.A.; Stillersfeld, J.M.; Wöstmann, B.; Schmidt, A. Update on the Accuracy of Conventional and Digital Full-Arch Impressions of Partially Edentulous and Fully Dentate Jaws in Young and Elderly Subjects: A Clinical Trial. *J. Clin. Med.* **2022**, *11*, 3723. https://doi.org/10.3390/jcm11133723

Academic Editors: Adolfo Di Fiore and Giulia Brunello

Received: 24 May 2022
Accepted: 25 June 2022
Published: 28 June 2022

Publisher's Note: MDPI stays neutral with regard to jurisdictional claims in published maps and institutional affiliations.

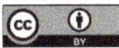

Copyright: © 2022 by the authors. Licensee MDPI, Basel, Switzerland. This article is an open access article distributed under the terms and conditions of the Creative Commons Attribution (CC BY) license (https://creativecommons.org/licenses/by/4.0/).

Abstract: To update the available literature on the accuracy of conventional and digital full-arch impressions using the latest hardware and software, participants of different age groups and dental status were investigated. An established reference aid-based method was applied to analyze five intraoral scanners (IOS) CS 3800 (CS), iTero Element 5D (IT), Medit i700 (ME), Primescan (PS), and Trios 4 (TR), and one conventional polyether impression (CVI). Forty-five participants were classified into three groups: Age 27.3 ± 2.7 years fully dentate, 60.6 ± 8.1 years fully dentate, and 65.7 ± 6.2 years partially edentulous. The IOS datasets were investigated using three-dimensional software (GOM Inspect), and plaster casts of CVI were analyzed using a co-ordinate measurement machine. The deviations of the reference aid to impressions were determined. No significant differences in age between the three groups were observed by the IOS in terms of trueness ($p < 0.05$). These findings were confirmed for precision, except for TR. In contrast to CS (mean ± standard deviation 98.9 ± 62.1 µm) and IT (89.0 ± 91.0 µm), TR (58.3 ± 66.8 µm), ME (57.9 ± 66.7 µm), and PS (55.5 ± 48.7 µm) did not show significant differences than those of CVI (34.8 ± 29.6 µm) in overall view. Within the study, the latest IOSs still showed limitations in the accuracy of full-arch impressions. However, they seemed to be unaffected by age and fully dentate or partially edentulous dentitions with small gaps.

Keywords: clinical study; intraoral scanners; digital dentistry; impression techniques; full-arch impression; elderly population; dimensional measurement accuracy

1. Introduction

To date, a physical or virtual model of the intraoral situation is required for any indirect restoration or dental appliances [1]. Therefore, several conventional and digital techniques are currently available for full-arch impressions [2]. However, for impression-taking in the aged population, data are scarce [3]. In contrast to young, fully dentate patients, who mostly require impressions for orthodontic appliances or night guards, tooth loss and prosthodontic restorations are expected with increasing patient age. Furthermore, the demographic change leads to an elderly population with patients presenting a high number of natural teeth due to preventive dental hygiene concepts [4,5]. Thus, dentists are facing an aging population with increasing fixed-dental restorations (FDP). This topic needs to be addressed urgently.

Even though the general requirements for accuracy according ISO 5725-1 (mean values describing trueness, standard deviation (SD) describing precision) [6] are precise representations of the intraoral situation and an exact transfer to the extraoral model in this context, aged dentitions often exhibit attachment loss of the soft tissue with gingival recession and extensive interdental areas in contrast to young, natural dentate jaws and therefore present the practitioner with increased challenges [7,8]. Apart from the physiological aging of dentitions, the high prevalence of periodontitis, up to 42% in patients aged 40–60 years and up to 68% in patients aged >65 years, is also a contributing factor [9,10]. The implications of severe periodontitis are tooth loss, pathologic tooth migration with malocclusion, and flaring or elongation of teeth with bite deepening [11–13]. In summary, several undercuts complicate accurate impression taking.

A previous clinical study revealed that digital impressions with intraoral scanners (IOS) are superior to conventional polyvinyl siloxane impressions concerning the ability to display interdental areas in periodontally compromised dentitions in the aged population [3]. This can be explained by tearing and distortion of the conventional impression material during the removal of the impression because the elastomeric material flows into the undercuts and sets. However, the accuracies of both digital and conventional impressions were not investigated. For the entire impression of areas with undercuts, the scanning tip of the IOS cannot be positioned parallel to the tooth surface, resulting in angulations of up to 45°. Whether this angulation may cause inaccuracy in intraoral scan datasets needs to be discussed. A laboratory study by Desoutter et al. [14] has described higher noise for the IOS datasets captured with angulated surfaces of 30° and 45° than that with plane surfaces without angulation. To the best of the authors' knowledge, no study has investigated the influence of aged dentition accompanied by further challenges on the accuracy of full-arch impressions.

Although clinical studies described superior accuracy for IOSs of short-span FDP within one quadrant compared to conventional impressions (CVIs), the latter still revealed the highest accuracy for long-span distances in the full-arch [15,16]. This is because the main problem with the IOS is that all scanning systems available in the market today do not allow an entire jaw or even just one-half of the jaw to be captured at once. All systems provide only sectional images covering a small area and must be merged by the scanner's software in a matching/stitching process to create an overall model of the complete jaw. Although the original accuracy of the scanners is very high in the systems currently available in the market, these matching algorithms determine how accurately the overall system of hardware and software can map the geometry of the jaw. Matching errors lead to a steady increase without a compensable total error as the reconstruction of the jaw progresses along the scan path [17]. This is a fundamental disadvantage of the digital impression technique compared to the conventional methods because the latter captures the jaw all at once. Further development of hardware and software in recent years has shown a constant improvement in the IOS; hence, the latest IOS generations might overcome this limitation [16,18]. However, for new IOSs, such as CS 3800 (Carestream Dental, Atlanta, GA, USA), iTero Element 5D (Align Technology, San José, CA, USA), and Medit i700 (Medit, Seoul, South Korea), no clinical data for the accuracy of full-arch impression have been published yet.

To assess the accuracy of different impression techniques, a reference aid that displays the actual patient's situation is indispensable [15]. Otherwise, only the respective deviations of different impression techniques can be examined. Only two reference aid-based methods have been described in the literature [19,20]. However, clinical data are only available for fully dentate jaws. Recently, Kontis et al. [21] published the first data on partially edentulous models based on a laboratory study with a reference aid, revealing a reduced accuracy compared to that of fully dentate models. In particular, edentulous areas in the mandible with mucosal mobility and saliva may be challenging in clinical impression taking.

Therefore, this clinical study aimed to update the available literature on the accuracy (trueness and precision according to ISO 5725 [6]) of conventional and digital full-arch impressions using the latest hardware and software in different age groups with partially edentulous and fully dentate mandibular jaws.

The null hypotheses investigated were as follows: there are no significant differences between young and elderly subjects in different clinical situations (I), and there are no significant differences among the six impression techniques investigated (II).

2. Materials and Methods

Forty-five participants were included in this clinical study and classified into three groups with different clinical situations as follows:

- Group A: Age 27.3 ± 2.7 years with fully dentate mandibular jaw (n = 15)
- Group B: Age 60.6 ± 8.1 years with fully dentate mandibular jaw (n = 15)
- Group C: Age 65.7 ± 6.2 years with partially edentulous mandibular jaw with unilateral edentulous space and adjacent natural teeth (Kennedy Class III, n = 15).

Good oral hygiene and stable positioning of the reference aid on the occlusal surfaces of the mandibular jaw were defined as further inclusion criteria. Participants with severe systemic disease, epilepsy, or allergies to the materials used were excluded. Furthermore, patients with attachments on tooth surface (e.g., orthodontic appliances) were not included. For a better overview, Figure 1 displays a flow scheme of the clinical trial.

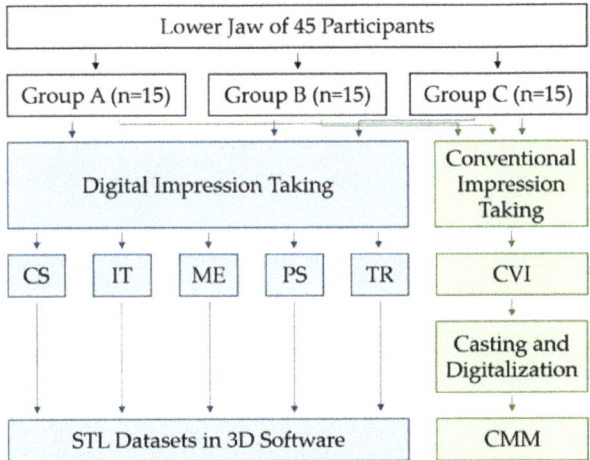

Figure 1. Flow scheme of the clinical trial (CS = CS 3800, IT = iTero Element 5D, ME = Medit i700, PS = Primescan, TR = Trios 4, CVI = conventional impression, STL = standard tessellation language, CMM = coordinate measuring machine).

To ensure comparable testing conditions, all experiments were performed by a single operator (J.M.S.) trained on conventional impression taking and all IOSs used in this study.

The investigations were conducted at the Department of Prosthodontics of the Justus Liebig University (JLU) Giessen, Germany, in full compliance with ethical principles, including the Declaration of Helsinki of the World Medical Association. The clinical study was approved by the local ethics committee of the JLU (Ref. no. 163/15) and recorded in the German Clinical Trial Register (DRKS00027135).

According to an established reference method previously described in the literature, four steel spheres (1.3505 100Cr6 DIN5401; TIS GmbH, Gauting, Germany; diameter, 5 mm; roundness, 5000 ± 5.63 µm [22]) were reversibly bonded to the mandibular teeth with a flowable composite (Grandio Flow, Voco, Cuxhaven, Germany) [16,20]. A metal reference guide (Bretthauer GmbH, Dillenburg, Germany; Figure 2) was used to position the spheres presenting a reproducible placement with a precision of <10 µm [23]. When the reference plate was removed, the spheres remained in a defined position, allowing subsequent comparison to the original position in the reference plate.

Before taking digital impressions with the IOS, calibration of the scanner tip with the respective calibration device was applied [24]. The established scan strategy—starting on the occlusal surface, followed by the oral surfaces, and finishing on the buccal surfaces—

as recommended by manufacturers was performed [3,16,21]. The IOS used with the corresponding software versions are listed in Table 1.

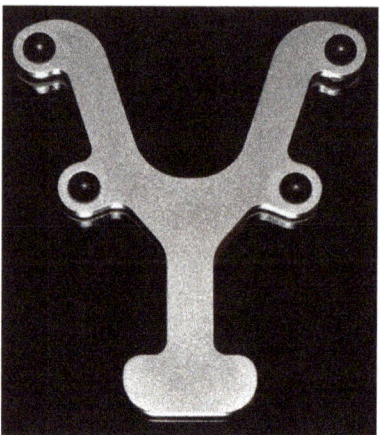

Figure 2. Metal reference guide with the four steel spheres inserted.

Table 1. Intraoral scanners used in this study.

Product Name	Manufacturer	Software Version	Abbreviation
CS 3800	Carestream Dental (Atlanta, GA, USA)	1.0.4	CS
iTero Element 5D	Align Technology (San José, CA, USA)	2.7.0.990	IT
Medit i700	Medit (Seoul, South Korea)	1.7.4	ME
Primescan	Dentsply Sirona (Bensheim, Germany)	5.1.3	PS
Trios 4 wireless POD	3Shape (Copenhagen, Denmark)	21.2.0	TR

Cheek retractors (Optragate, Ivoclar Vivadent, Schaan, Lichtenstein) and dry tips (Microbrush International, Grafton, WI, USA) were placed intraorally to control the soft tissue and saliva. Furthermore, uniform light conditions were applied during digital impression taking [25]. For each subject, one scan was performed. Scan data were exported as standard tessellation language (STL) datasets. After completing the digital impressions, the cheek retractor and dry tips were removed, and a CVI was obtained using medium-weight polyether impression material (Impregum Penta Soft Quick, batch number 4811262, 3M Espe, Minneapolis, MN, USA) and a standard metal tray (Ehricke stainless steel, Orbis Dental, Münster, Germany). Before casting with type IV dental stone (Fujirock EP, batch number 1810031, GC Corporation, Tokyo, Japan), the CVI was stored for at least 2 h to ensure elastic recovery.

Plaster casts were stored under laboratory conditions (temperature 23 ± 1 °C; humidity 50 ± 10%) for at least 5 days before measurement. To measure the reference and plaster models, a co-ordinate measuring machine (CMM, Thome Präzision GmbH, Messel, Germany) with the corresponding software (X4 V10 GA ×64, Metrologic Group, Meylan, France) was used. For the reference dataset the spheres were inserted into the reference aid, measured 10 times with the CMM, and the mean value for each sphere position was calculated. The resulting digital reference model was saved in IGES (Initial Graphics Exchange Specification) format. Subsequently, plaster models of CVIs were also measured with the CMM and saved as digital datasets. The STL datasets of the digital impressions were imported into a three-dimensional analysis software (GOM Inspect 2019, v2.0.1, gom, Braunschweig, Germany). Then, the linear distances between the centers of the spheres were determined (Figure 3).

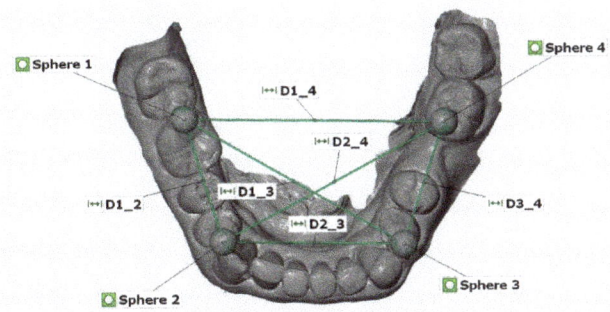

Figure 3. Example of the measurement of linear distances (D1_2, D1_3, D1_4, D2_3, D2_4, D3_4) between the centers of the four spheres 1–4 (top view of STL dataset in GOM software).

To measure the deviations between the reference dataset and the models, the reference dataset of the reference aid was imported and saved as computer-aided design data in the analysis program. The scans were imported as an STL dataset and saved as the actual data. Then, fitting elements (Gauss best fit, 3 sigma) were used to construct the sphere elements on the scanned spheres. Subsequently, deviations between the measured distances of the intraoral scans and the reference guide were calculated.

Statistical analysis was performed using the SPSS software (version 28, IBM, Armonk, NY, USA). For trueness [6], the data were transformed using a square root transformation. A three-factor analysis of variance (ANOVA) was performed with the factors' impression, distance, and dentition. Because impression and distance are repeated factors, dependencies arose, which were considered by a variance component model (procedure MIXED). Distance and impression were modeled as repeated-measures factors; therefore, variance heterogeneity resulting from these factors was also considered. To account for this variance heterogeneity, the three factors were modeled as repeated measurements. The decision criterion was the p-value of the interaction, followed by that of the model comparison using -2LL-chi-squared tests. Pairwise comparisons of the hypotheses were requested via the estimated marginal means (margins) and corrected with the Bonferroni correction for multiple pairwise tests. For a better overview, the data are presented in boxplots. For precision, the scatter of different factor levels was tested for homogeneity. Pairwise Levene tests were used to compare impressions within and between groups with respect to distance. To account for the dependencies in the data due to multiple measurements, tests were performed using model residuals. The tests were performed on model residuals from the mixed linear models. The robust Levene tests were based on the medians (Brown–Forsythe test). Differences with $p < 0.05$ were considered statistically significant.

3. Results

The overall results with pooled data of linear distances for the six impression techniques classified into three groups A, B, and C, are displayed in Figure 4.

Regarding participants' age, no significant differences between the three groups were observed for IOS in terms of trueness. These findings were confirmed with respect to precision, except for Trios 4, with significant differences between groups A/B and B/C. In contrast to the IOS, the CVI showed significant differences between groups A/B and B/C for trueness and between groups B/C for precision. Table 2 reports the pairwise comparisons for different groups and impression techniques.

Concerning the impression technique, no significant difference was observed between the IOSs ME, PS, and TR compared to the CVI in the overall view. However, the CVI still showed the lowest deviation, especially with respect to long-span distances. The two IOSs, CS and IT, exhibited the highest deviations.

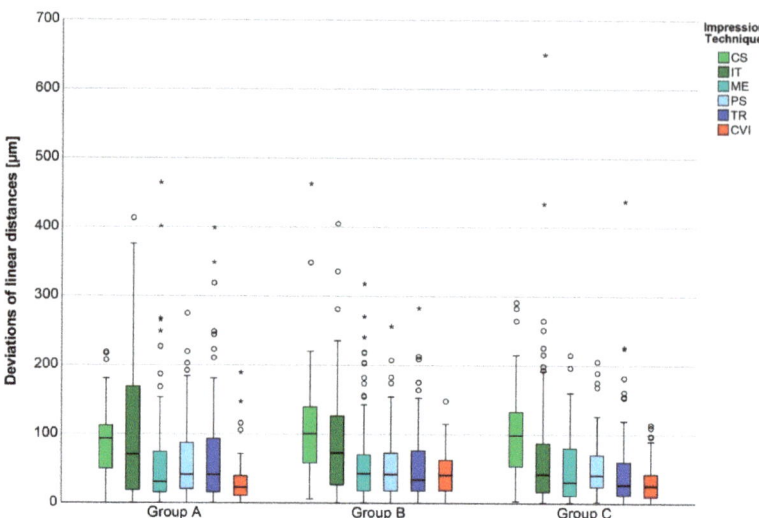

Figure 4. Boxplot diagram of pooled data of the deviations of linear distances for the six impression techniques (CS = CS 3800, IT = iTero Element 5D, ME = Medit i700, PS = Primescan, TR = Trios 4, CVI = conventional impression) classified to group A, B, and C; outliners (O), extreme values (*).

Table 2. Deviations (mean ± standard deviation (SD) [μm]) of the pooled data of linear distances (D1_2, D1_3, D1_4, D2_3, D2_4, D3_4) of six impression techniques (CS = CS 3800, IT = iTero Element 5D, ME = Medit i700, PS = Primescan, TR = Trios 4, CVI = conventional impression) for all groups and statistical analysis for trueness (upper right part) and precision (lower left part, presented in bold type) according to ISO 5725 [6].

Impression Technique	Group	Mean (Trueness) ± SD (Precision) [μm]	Group A	Group B	Group C
CS	A	87.1 ± 51.6	-	0.237	0.533
	B	107.3 ± 71.1	**0.374**	-	>0.999
	C	102.2 ± 60.8	**0.108**	**0.639**	-
IT	A	101.5 ± 97.1	-	>0.999	0.784
	B	90.5 ± 78.3	**0.118**	-	0.502
	C	75.0 ± 96.4	**0.986**	**0.163**	-
ME	A	61.5 ± 81.7	-	0.881	>0.999
	B	62.2 ± 66.0	**0.695**	-	0.314
	C	49.9 ± 48.4	**0.187**	**0.295**	-
PS	A	60.7 ± 55.1	-	0.649	>0.999
	B	53.6 ± 49.6	**0.302**	-	>0.999
	C	52.2 ± 40.4	**0.475**	**0.723**	-
TR	A	69.4 ± 79.3	-	>0.999	0.814
	B	55.0 ± 53.4	**0.013**	-	>0.999
	C	50.6 ± 64.3	**0.746**	**0.041**	-
CVI	A	30.5 ± 31.2	-	0.012	>0.999
	B	43.5 ± 30.4	**0.179**	-	0.020
	C	30.3 ± 25.3	**0.397**	**0.009**	-

However, the highest linear deviations were still observed for long-span distances across all the IOSs. Even though the overall results did not show any significant difference in terms of trueness and only a few regarding precision, the detailed analysis of the linear distances exhibited isolated significant differences for accuracy in groups A, B, and C (Figure 5).

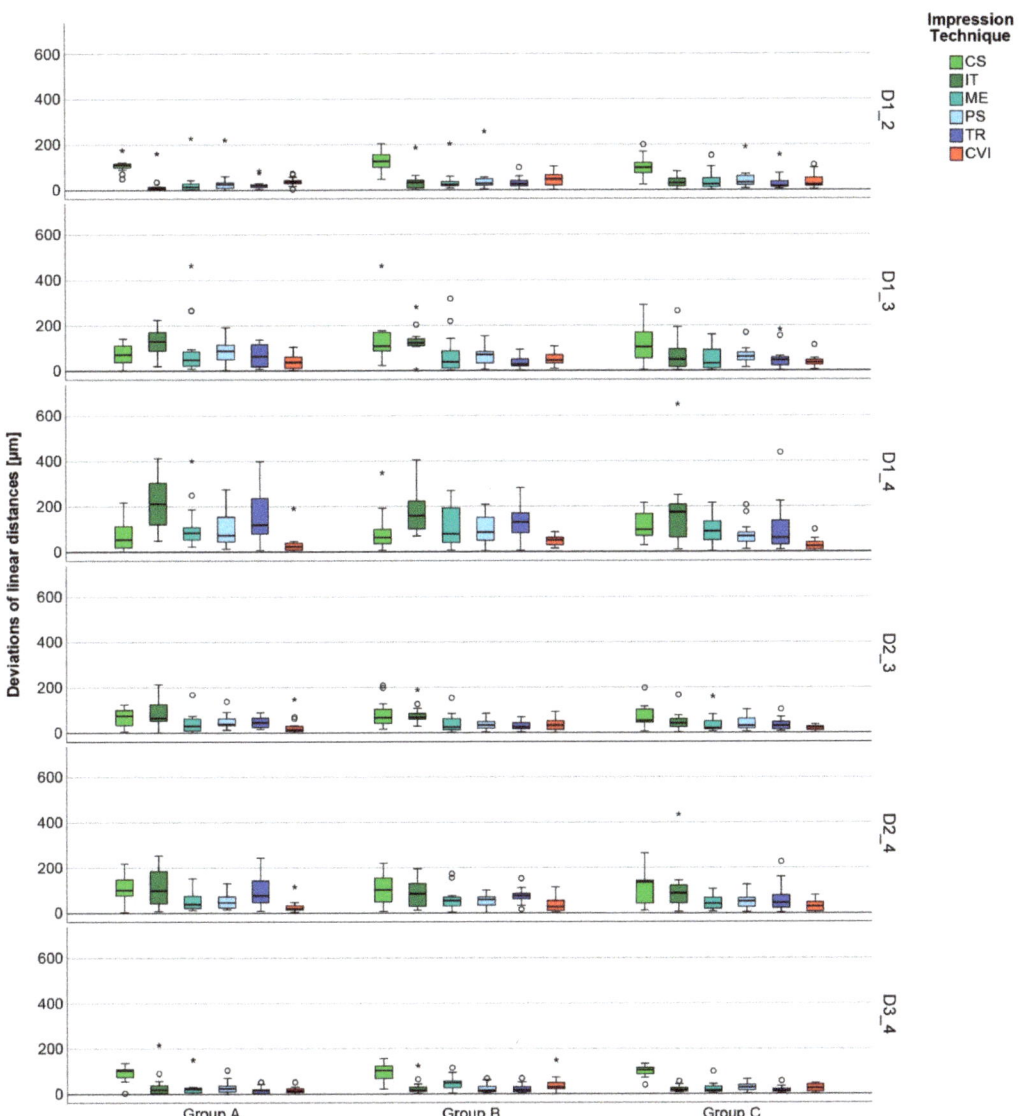

Figure 5. Boxplot diagram of the deviations of the linear distances (D1_2, D1_3, D1_4, D2_3, D2_4, D3_4) in group A, B, and C for the six techniques (CS = CS 3800, IT = iTero Element 5D, ME = Medit i700, PS = Primescan, TR = Trios 4, CVI = conventional impression); outliners (o), extreme values (*).

Regarding group A, isolated significant differences were observed between the different IOSs for all distances for trueness. In contrast, only considerably fewer significant deviations occurred with precision.

In group B, isolated significant differences between the individual IOSs with respect to distances in terms of trueness were observed as well. In terms of precision, less significant differences were observed between the individual IOSs.

Isolated significant differences between the individual IOSs with respect to distances in terms of trueness were noted in group C. In terms of precision, less significant differences were observed between the individual IOSs. The detailed values are presented in the Appendix A (Tables A1–A3).

Partly significant differences with respect to young and elderly subjects, clinical situations, and different impression techniques were noted; hence, both null hypotheses were rejected.

4. Discussion

In previous studies, numerous influencing factors have been identified with regard to digital impression taking [26]. Thus, the most recent software versions of the respective IOS were used [27–29]. Furthermore, all IOSs were calibrated before each impression was taken according to the manufacturer's instructions to avoid possible deviations [24]. In addition, measurements were conducted with a reference structure [16,20,23] that allows one to determine trueness and precision [15,19]. This allowed the measurement of the individual linear distances and their possible distance deviations across the entire jaw.

As different scanning paths can lead to different results, the scanning path recommended by the manufacturers was used [30,31]. To avoid the influence of different examiners, all impressions were obtained by a trained operator [32]. Due to the methodology used of the reference plate, only impressions of the mandibular jaw were investigated, and this may be regarded as a limitation.

Previous studies addressing the accuracy have typically examined eugnathia dentitions [15,16,20]. However, the dental status and mucosal situation changes with age. Particularly, the mucosal situation in older patients is different from that in young patients. This is directly related to the increase in undercuts and root surfaces being exposed with advancing age on the remaining teeth in the oral cavity [7,8]. To date, only one clinical study has investigated impressions of periodontal compromised dentitions [3]. The increase in the number of undercuts on natural teeth is particularly important for both conventional and digital impressions. While conventional impressions allow the impression material to flow into the undercuts, which typically tear off during removal, high tear strength is often relied upon when selecting the material [33]. However, digital impressions seem to show a clear advantage over conventional impressions, and undercuts also present a particular challenge for the acquisition of a digital impression through the IOS. Because IOSs can only record data in the scanning field, the scanner's handpiece must be rotated into the undercuts to detect them as well [3,34]. For this reason, aged dentitions, especially ones with undercuts, make it challenging for the practitioner and the impression method used to obtain high accuracies with regard to the transfer of the intraoral to the model situation.

This is also aggravated by matching and stitching errors predominantly occurring in digital impression taking when long distances and edentulous areas are recorded. Therefore, it was anticipated that dentitions with gaps show higher inaccuracies in contrast to fully dentate jaws because the respective teeth, which typically serve as references, are missing. The comparison of the results of the present study to data in the literature was difficult, since, to our knowledge, only one in vitro study by Kontis et al. [21] has been conducted to date regarding the accuracy of the IOS with missing teeth and a reference structure. It should be noted, however, that owing to the different design of the study (bar versus spheres), only the intermolar distance of the present study could be used for direct comparison.

Regarding the deviations of the individual scanners in the respective groups, significant differences were only found for Trios 4 with regard to precision and CVI with regard to both trueness and precision. The precision of Trios 4 was the lowest in group A. However, compared to Kontis et al. [21], lower deviations were obtained in the present study with Primescan. This might be attributed to the different evaluation and reference methods used. The high inaccuracies of gap situations described by Kontis et al. are supposed to be related to wider gaps, which foster matching or stitching errors [17,19,20,23,35].

However, the results of CVI in the present study could be compared with those in previous studies with the same methodology [16,20]. The results of Trios 4 and Primescan are comparable to a previous study as well [16].

Keul and Güth have used an older version of the iTero IOS [15]. The slightly better results shown by Keul and Güth are supposed to be related on the references bar, which allows a better overlay of the individual datasets. Additionally, in contrast to the investigation by Keul and Güth [15], this study used mandibular jaws. In contrast to the upper jaws and even an in vitro experiment, greater deviations due to the saliva, reflections, and movements of the subjects were expected in the mandibular jaw. Nevertheless, this type of study reflects daily practice since the clinical framework conditions pose challenges to every practitioner.

Unfortunately, currently, no comparable data for the current IOS CS 3800, iTero Element 5D, and Medit i700 exist, which makes it difficult to compare the available results. What was striking in the comparison, however, was that the CS 3800, in contrast to all other IOSs, displayed comparably higher inaccuracies, especially for short distances, regardless of the group.

For CVI, groups A and C did not differ significantly in terms of trueness. In contrast, group B showed greater deviations. However, these were still the smallest compared to the digital impressions. In terms of precision, this was only the case between groups B and C. In principle, the results of the conventional impression could be directly compared to the results of the previous study with regard to group A [16]. A lower trueness in group B was noticeable. This group of subjects with older dentition situations showed the undercuts exactly where possible tear-out distortions could lead to higher deviations. This would also explain the higher trueness in group C, as lower removal forces were necessary when removing the impressions with lower residual tooth stock, which could correlate to lower stresses within the material in connection with the lower necessity of the restoring forces [36].

In summary, only one IOS showed a difference among the different age groups in terms of accuracy. Significant differences were observed only in the CVI. Follow-up studies with participants of an increasingly older population and not limited to young individuals are necessary.

5. Conclusions

Within the limitations of this study, we concluded that the latest IOSs still showed limitations in the accuracy of full-arch impressions, even though they all revealed a mean of less than 100 μm deviations on overall view. Furthermore, it has to be noticed that there are still significant differences between the various IOSs. However, they seemed to be unaffected by age and fully dentate or partially edentulous dentitions with small gaps.

Author Contributions: Conceptualization, M.A.S. and A.S.; methodology, M.A.S., B.W. and A.S.; software, A.S.; validation, M.A.S., B.W. and A.S.; formal analysis, A.S.; investigation, J.M.S.; resources, B.W.; data curation, M.A.S., J.M.S. and A.S.; writing—original draft preparation, M.A.S. and A.S.; writing—review and editing, B.W.; visualization, M.A.S.; supervision, M.A.S. and A.S.; project administration, M.A.S.; funding acquisition, M.A.S. and B.W. All authors have read and agreed to the published version of the manuscript.

Funding: This research was conducted with the support of SIRONA Dental Systems GmbH.

Institutional Review Board Statement: The study was conducted according to the guidelines of the Declaration of Helsinki and was approved by the Ethics Committee of the Justus Liebig University Giessen (Ref. no. 163/15).

Informed Consent Statement: Informed consent was obtained from all subjects involved in the study.

Data Availability Statement: The datasets in this article are available from the corresponding author upon a reasonable request.

Acknowledgments: The authors would like to thank the dental company SIRONA Dental Systems GmbH for supporting this study. Furthermore, we gratefully acknowledge the support of our biostatistician, Johannes Herrmann, for the statistical analysis.

Conflicts of Interest: The authors declare no conflict of interest.

Appendix A

Table A1. Deviations (mean ± standard deviation (SD) [µm]) of the linear distances (D1_2, D1_3, D1_4, D2_3, D2_4, D3_4) of six impression techniques (CS = CS 3800, IT = iTero Element 5D, ME = Medit i700, PS = Primescan, TR = Trios 4, CVI = conventional impression) for Group A (young fully dentate) and statistical analysis for trueness (upper right part) and precision (lower left part, presented in bold type) according to ISO 5725 [6].

Linear Distances	Impression Technique	Mean (Trueness) ± SD (Precision) [µm]	CS	IT	ME	PS	TR	CVI
D1_2	CS	110.9 ± 32.2	-	<0.001	<0.001	<0.001	<0.001	<0.001
	IT	21.2 ± 39.8	**0.682**	-	>0.999	>0.999	>0.999	>0.999
	ME	30.3 ± 56.2	**0.583**	**0.797**	-	>0.999	>0.999	>0.999
	PS	35.6 ± 53.5	**0.199**	**0.330**	**0.528**	-	>0.999	>0.999
	TR	25.0 ± 23.5	**0.399**	**0.321**	**0.353**	**0.108**	-	>0.999
	CVI	37.0 ± 18.1	**0.639**	**0.462**	**0.452**	**0.142**	**0.628**	-
D1_3	CS	73.7 ± 47.6	-	>0.999	0.186	>0.999	0.017	<0.001
	IT	125.9 ± 62.8	**0.393**	-	0.002	0.067	<0.001	<0.001
	ME	100.5 ± 130.2	**0.080**	**0.142**	-	>0.999	>0.999	>0.999
	PS	87.4 ± 50.2	**0.214**	**0.470**	**0.329**	-	0.221	<0.001
	TR	67.4 ± 49.7	**0.455**	**0.842**	**0.121**	**0.386**	-	>0.999
	CVI	37.9 ± 31.4	**0.626**	**0.225**	**0.061**	**0.144**	**0.247**	-
D1_4	CS	75.3 ± 69.6	-	<0.001	>0.999	>0.999	0.300	<0.001
	IT	219.9 ± 116.9	**0.098**	-	<0.001	<0.001	0.242	<0.001
	ME	110.5 ± 100.4	**0.343**	**0.518**	-	>0.999	>0.999	<0.001
	PS	104.1 ± 76.4	**0.323**	**0.021**	**0.102**	-	0.823	<0.001
	TR	163.9 ± 122.9	**0.367**	**0.306**	**0.781**	**0.054**	-	<0.001
	CVI	33.2 ± 46.0	**0.010**	**0.002**	**0.009**	**0.031**	**<0.001**	-
D2_3	CS	64.7 ± 40.5	-	>0.999	0.095	>0.999	0.227	<0.001
	IT	88.8 ± 56.7	**0.331**	-	0.011	0.176	0.022	<0.001
	ME	42.1 ± 42.8	**0.554**	**0.539**	-	>0.999	>0.999	0.379
	PS	51.4 ± 33.4	**0.274**	**0.123**	**0.108**	-	>0.999	0.001
	TR	47.5 ± 24.6	**0.117**	**0.882**	**0.291**	**0.018**	-	0.006
	CVI	28.9 ± 38.8	**0.154**	**0.090**	**0.054**	**0.773**	**0.009**	-
D2_4	CS	108.6 ± 64.3	-	>0.999	0.009	0.044	>0.999	<0.001
	IT	116.9 ± 83.3	**0.058**	-	0.022	0.084	>0.999	<0.001
	ME	51.9 ± 39.0	**0.810**	**0.046**	-	>0.999	0.098	0.023
	PS	55.8 ± 38.9	**0.167**	**0.005**	**0.316**	-	0.402	0.002
	TR	95.8 ± 71.9	**0.469**	**0.195**	**0.368**	**0.048**	-	<0.001
	CVI	29.1 ± 27.4	**0.022**	**<0.001**	**0.063**	**0.224**	**0.006**	-
D3_4	CS	89.5 ± 32.1	-	<0.001	<0.001	<0.001	<0.001	<0.001
	IT	36.3 ± 55.1	**0.028**	-	>0.999	>0.999	>0.999	>0.999
	ME	33.6 ± 48.3	**0.015**	**0.918**	-	>0.999	>0.999	>0.999
	PS	30.1 ± 29.2	**0.006**	**0.313**	**0.236**	-	>0.999	>0.999
	TR	16.5 ± 16.1	**0.041**	**0.913**	**0.829**	**0.389**	-	>0.999
	CVI	16.9 ± 13.6	**<0.001**	**0.823**	**0.913**	**0.093**	**0.727**	-

Table A2. Deviations (mean ± standard deviation (SD) [μm]) of the linear distances (D1_2, D1_3, D1_4, D2_3, D2_4, D3_4) of six impression techniques (CS = CS 3800, IT = iTero Element 5D, ME = Medit i700, PS = Primescan, TR = Trios 4, CVI = conventional impression) for Group B (young fully dentate) and statistical analysis for trueness (upper right part) and precision (lower left part, presented in bold type) according to ISO 5725 [6].

Linear Distances	Impression Technique	Mean (Trueness) ± SD (Precision) [μm]	CS	IT	ME	PS	TR	CVI
D1_2	CS	127.8 ± 46.4	-	<0.001	<0.001	<0.001	<0.001	<0.001
	IT	36.3 ± 45.7	0.169	-	>0.999	<0.001	>0.999	0.164
	ME	37.7 ± 48.3	0.151	0.898	-	>0.999	>0.999	0.700
	PS	44.4 ± 61.2	0.432	0.898	0.833	-	>0.999	0.461
	TR	31.7 ± 24.8	<0.001	0.003	0.010	0.083	-	0.004
	CVI	47.3 ± 33.5	0.059	0.637	0.756	0.672	0.005	-
D1_3	CS	137.2 ± 100.7	-	>0.999	0.079	0.038	<0.001	<0.001
	IT	132.1 ± 57.9	0.129	-	0.011	0.003	<0.001	<0.001
	ME	72.2 ± 91.4	0.897	0.124	-	>0.999	>0.999	>0.999
	PS	66.3 ± 45.5	0.263	0.511	0.277	-	0.508	>0.999
	TR	36.6 ± 29.2	0.041	0.416	0.030	0.099	-	>0.999
	CVI	51.0 ± 28.2	0.036	0.354	0.026	0.082	0.775	-
D1_4	CS	89.1 ± 88.0	-	<0.001	>0.999	>0.999	>0.999	<0.001
	IT	180.3 ± 95.5	0.621	-	0.004	<0.001	0.059	<0.001
	ME	114.2 ± 87.4	0.565	0.904	-	>0.999	>0.999	<0.001
	PS	97.5 ± 63.7	0.107	0.012	0.018	-	0.362	0.018
	TR	131.6 ± 72.9	0.099	0.010	0.016	0.932	-	<0.001
	CVI	47.7 ± 22.5	0.017	<0.001	0.002	0.026	0.028	-
D2_3	CS	85.3 ± 57.8	-	>0.999	0.028	0.001	<0.001	<0.001
	IT	79.1 ± 39.5	0.260	-	0.041	0.002	<0.001	>0.999
	ME	40.4 ± 41.4	0.511	0.617	-	>0.999	>0.999	<0.001
	PS	37.4 ± 26.0	0.012	0.244	0.067	-	>0.999	>0.999
	TR	30.5 ± 20.5	0.025	0.383	0.125	0.468	-	>0.999
	CVI	36.7 ± 28.5	0.085	0.737	0.326	0.104	0.312	-
D2_4	CS	107.3 ± 68.6	-	>0.999	0.003	<0.001	0.201	<0.001
	IT	88.3 ± 61.3	0.863	-	0.111	0.005	>0.999	<0.001
	ME	62.2 ± 47.2	0.984	0.876	-	>0.999	>0.999	0.651
	PS	52.7 ± 32.7	0.005	0.008	0.004	-	0.099	>0.999
	TR	76.6 ± 33.0	<0.001	<0.001	<0.001	0.085	-	0.005
	CVI	38.3 ± 33.6	0.006	0.009	0.005	0.972	0.088	-
D3_4	CS	96.9 ± 40.7	-	<0.001	<0.001	<0.001	<0.001	<0.001
	IT	26.8 ± 31.6	0.459	-	>0.999	>0.999	>0.999	>0.999
	ME	46.2 ± 31.2	0.323	0.112	-	0.860	0.045	>0.999
	PS	23.0 ± 19.9	0.371	0.994	0.064	-	>0.999	>0.999
	TR	22.9 ± 19.3	0.001	0.043	<0.001	0.003	-	0.060
	CVI	39.8 ± 36.2	0.298	0.803	0.060	0.758	0.062	-

Table A3. Deviations (mean ± standard deviation (SD) [μm]) of the linear distances (D1_2, D1_3, D1_4, D2_3, D2_4, D3_4) of six impression techniques (CS = CS 3800, IT = iTero Element 5D, ME = Medit i700, PS = Primescan, TR = Trios 4, CVI = conventional impression) for Group C (young fully dentate) and statistical analysis for trueness (upper right part) and precision (lower left part, presented in bold type) according to ISO 5725 [6].

Linear Distances	Impression Technique	Mean (Trueness) ± SD (Precision) [μm]	CS	IT	ME	PS	TR	CVI
D1_2	CS	101.0 ± 47.7	-	<0.001	<0.001	<0.001	<0.001	<0.001
	IT	34.4 ± 23.8	0.320	-	>0.999	>0.999	>0.999	0.760

Table A3. Cont.

Linear Distances	Impression Technique	Mean (Trueness) ± SD (Precision) [μm]	p-Value					
			CS	IT	ME	PS	TR	CVI
D1_2	ME	41.2 ± 43.9	0.761	0.364	-	>0.999	>0.999	>0.999
	PS	46.2 ± 44.8	0.722	0.369	0.946	-	>0.999	>0.999
	TR	32.5 ± 39.4	0.020	0.248	0.097	0.118	-	0.795
	CVI	38.8 ± 34.8	0.784	0.370	0.975	0.922	0.094	-
D1_3	CS	120.8 ± 88.1	-	>0.999	0.007	0.215	<0.001	<0.001
	IT	73.4 ± 78.5	0.657	-	0.007	0.197	<0.001	<0.001
	ME	52.8 ± 51.9	0.588	0.942	-	>0.999	>0.999	>0.999
	PS	66.1 ± 37.3	0.004	0.024	0.018	-	0.063	0.001
	TR	51.9 ± 51.5	0.149	0.340	0.353	0.196	-	>0.999
	CVI	38.1 ± 26.1	<0.001	0.006	0.004	0.196	0.062	-
D1_4	CS	111.5 ± 60.3	-	0.003	>0.999	>0.999	>0.999	<0.001
	IT	170.7 ± 154.8	0.181	-	0.003	<0.001	0.309	<0.001
	ME	91.9 ± 64.8	0.162	0.693	-	>0.999	>0.999	<0.001
	PS	76.1 ± 53.2	0.428	0.073	0.030	-	>0.999	<0.001
	TR	102.1 ± 112.0	0.464	0.454	0.610	0.167	-	<0.001
	CVI	29.0 ± 25.7	0.011	0.010	<0.001	0.020	0.010	-
D2_3	CS	70.0 ± 48.9	-	>0.999	<0.001	0.020	<0.001	<0.001
	IT	48.3 ± 39.8	0.925	-	0.025	0.407	0.019	<0.001
	ME	40.1 ± 40.5	0.903	0.837	-	>0.999	>0.999	0.795
	PS	41.2 ± 32.0	0.036	0.035	0.083	-	>0.999	0.005
	TR	35.9 ± 26.3	0.034	0.034	0.081	0.995	-	0.089
	CVI	19.5 ± 11.2	0.001	0.002	0.007	0.052	0.042	-
D2_4	CS	110.5 ± 72.0	-	>0.999	<0.001	<0.001	0.279	<0.001
	IT	102.2 ± 101.5	0.646	-	0.056	0.184	>0.999	<0.001
	ME	47.7 ± 33.2	0.591	0.381	-	>0.999	0.215	0.117
	PS	53.4 ± 35.4	0.011	0.026	0.006	-	0.729	0.016
	TR	63.6 ± 61.8	0.256	0.196	0.438	0.051	-	<0.001
	CVI	31.5 ± 27.9	<0.001	0.004	<0.001	0.013	<0.001	-
D3_4	CS	99.2 ± 24.7	-	<0.001	<0.001	<0.001	<0.001	<0.001
	IT	20.9 ± 13.5	0.430	-	>0.999	>0.999	>0.999	>0.999
	ME	25.8 ± 24.2	0.438	0.909	-	>0.999	0.509	>0.999
	PS	30.0 ± 19.4	0.014	0.142	0.252	-	0.304	>0.999
	TR	17.3 ± 14.0	0.334	0.118	0.166	0.001	-	>0.999
	CVI	24.9 ± 17.2	0.010	0.008	0.026	<0.001	0.051	-

References

1. Wöstmann, B. Abformmaterialien. In *Werkstoffkunde in der Zahnmedizin*; Rosentritt, M., Ilie, N., Lohbauer, U., Eds.; Thieme Verlag: Stuttgart, Germany, 2018; pp. 23–54.
2. Mangano, F.; Gandolfi, A.; Luongo, G.; Logozzo, S. Intraoral scanners in dentistry: A review of the current literature. *BMC Oral Health* **2017**, *17*, 149. [CrossRef] [PubMed]
3. Schlenz, M.A.; Schubert, V.; Schmidt, A.; Wöstmann, B.; Ruf, S.; Klaus, K. Digital versus Conventional Impression Taking Focusing on Interdental Areas: A Clinical Trial. *Int. J. Environ. Res. Public Health* **2020**, *17*, 4725. [CrossRef] [PubMed]
4. Jordan, R.A.; Bodechtel, C.; Hertrampf, K.; Hoffmann, T.; Kocher, T.; Nitschke, I.; Schiffner, U.; Stark, H.; Zimmer, S.; Micheelis, W.; et al. The Fifth German Oral Health Study (Funfte Deutsche Mundgesundheitsstudie, DMS V)—Rationale, design, and methods. *BMC Oral Health* **2014**, *14*, 161. [CrossRef]
5. Carlsson, G.E.; Omar, R. Trends in prosthodontics. *Med. Princ. Pract.* **2006**, *15*, 167–179. [CrossRef] [PubMed]
6. ISO 5725-1:1994; Accuracy (Trueness and Precision) of Measurement Methods and Results—Part 1: General Principles and Definitions. International Organization for Standardization: Geneva, Switzerland, 1994; pp. 1–17.
7. Heasman, P.A.; Ritchie, M.; Asuni, A.; Gavillet, E.; Simonsen, J.L.; Nyvad, B. Gingival recession and root caries in the ageing population: A critical evaluation of treatments. *J. Clin. Periodontol.* **2017**, *44* (Suppl. S18), S178–S193. [CrossRef]
8. McKenna, G.; Burke, F.M. Age-related oral changes. *Dent. Update* **2010**, *37*, 519–523. [CrossRef]
9. Demmer, R.T.; Papapanou, P.N. Epidemiologic patterns of chronic and aggressive periodontitis. *Periodontol 2000* **2010**, *53*, 28–44. [CrossRef]

10. Eke, P.I.; Wei, L.; Borgnakke, W.S.; Thornton-Evans, G.; Zhang, X.; Lu, H.; McGuire, L.C.; Genco, R.J. Periodontitis prevalence in adults >/= 65 years of age, in the USA. *Periodontol 2000* **2016**, *72*, 76–95. [CrossRef]
11. Martinez-Canut, P.; Carrasquer, A.; Magan, R.; Lorca, A. A study on factors associated with pathologic tooth migration. *J. Clin. Periodontol.* **1997**, *24*, 492–497. [CrossRef]
12. Brunsvold, M.A. Pathologic tooth migration. *J. Periodontol.* **2005**, *76*, 859–866. [CrossRef]
13. Melsen, B. *Adult Orthodontics*; Wiley-Blackwell Chichester: Hoboken, NJ, USA, 2012.
14. Desoutter, A.; Yusuf Solieman, O.; Subsol, G.; Tassery, H.; Cuisinier, F.; Fages, M. Method to evaluate the noise of 3D intra-oral scanner. *PLoS ONE* **2017**, *12*, e0182206. [CrossRef] [PubMed]
15. Keul, C.; Güth, J.F. Accuracy of full-arch digital impressions: An in vitro and in vivo comparison. *Clin. Oral Investig.* **2020**, *24*, 735–745. [CrossRef] [PubMed]
16. Schmidt, A.; Klussmann, L.; Wöstmann, B.; Schlenz, M.A. Accuracy of Digital and Conventional Full-Arch Impressions in Patients: An Update. *J. Clin. Med.* **2020**, *9*, 688. [CrossRef] [PubMed]
17. Schmidt, A.; Billig, J.W.; Schlenz, M.A.; Wöstmann, B. The Influence of Using Different Types of Scan Bodies on the Transfer Accuracy of Implant Position: An In Vitro Study. *Int. J. Prosthodont.* **2021**, *34*, 254–260. [CrossRef] [PubMed]
18. Giachetti, L.; Sarti, C.; Cinelli, F.; Russo, D.S. Accuracy of Digital Impressions in Fixed Prosthodontics: A Systematic Review of Clinical Studies. *Int. J. Prosthodont.* **2020**, *33*, 192–201. [CrossRef]
19. Güth, J.F.; Edelhoff, D.; Schweiger, J.; Keul, C. A new method for the evaluation of the accuracy of full-arch digital impressions in vitro. *Clin. Oral Investig.* **2016**, *20*, 1487–1494. [CrossRef]
20. Kuhr, F.; Schmidt, A.; Rehmann, P.; Wöstmann, B. A new method for assessing the accuracy of full arch impressions in patients. *J. Dent.* **2016**, *55*, 68–74. [CrossRef]
21. Kontis, P.; Guth, J.F.; Keul, C. Accuracy of full-arch digitalization for partially edentulous jaws—A laboratory study on basis of coordinate-based data analysis. *Clin. Oral Investig.* **2022**, *26*, 3651–3662. [CrossRef]
22. ISO 3290-1; Rolling Bearings—Balls—Part I: Steel Balls. International Organization for Standardization: Geneva, Switzerland, 2014.
23. Schmidt, A.; Klussmann, L.; Schlenz, M.A.; Wostmann, B. Elastic deformation of the mandibular jaw revisited-a clinical comparison between digital and conventional impressions using a reference. *Clin. Oral Investig.* **2021**, *25*, 4635–4642. [CrossRef]
24. Rehmann, P.; Sichwardt, V.; Wöstmann, B. Intraoral Scanning Systems: Need for Maintenance. *Int. J. Prosthodont.* **2017**, *30*, 27–29. [CrossRef]
25. Arakida, T.; Kanazawa, M.; Iwaki, M.; Suzuki, T.; Minakuchi, S. Evaluating the influence of ambient light on scanning trueness, precision, and time of intra oral scanner. *J. Prosthodont. Res.* **2018**, *62*, 324–329. [CrossRef] [PubMed]
26. Abduo, J.; Elseyoufi, M. Accuracy of Intraoral Scanners: A Systematic Review of Influencing Factors. *Eur. J. Prosthodont. Restor. Dent.* **2018**, *26*, 101–121. [CrossRef] [PubMed]
27. Schmidt, A.; Schlenz, M.A.; Liu, H.; Kämpe, H.S.; Wöstmann, B. The Influence of Hard- and Software Improvement of Intraoral Scanners on the Implant Transfer Accuracy from 2012 to 2021: An In Vitro Study. *Appl. Sci.* **2021**, *11*, 7166. [CrossRef]
28. Logozzo, S.; Zanetti, E.M.; Franceschini, G.; Kilpelä, A.; Mäkynen, A. Recent advances in dental optics—Part I: 3D intraoral scanners for restorative dentistry. *Opt. Lasers Eng.* **2014**, *54*, 203–221. [CrossRef]
29. Schmidt, A.; Benedickt, C.R.; Schlenz, M.A.; Rehmann, P.; Wostmann, B. Torsion and linear accuracy in intraoral scans obtained with different scanning principles. *J. Prosthodont. Res.* **2020**, *64*, 167–174. [CrossRef]
30. Ender, A.; Mehl, A. Influence of scanning strategies on the accuracy of digital intraoral scanning systems. *Int. J. Comput. Dent.* **2013**, *16*, 11–21.
31. Müller, P.; Ender, A.; Joda, T.; Katsoulis, J. Impact of digital intraoral scan strategies on the impression accuracy using the TRIOS Pod scanner. *Quintessence Int.* **2016**, *47*, 343–349. [CrossRef]
32. Resende, C.C.D.; Barbosa, T.A.Q.; Moura, G.F.; Tavares, L.D.N.; Rizzante, F.A.P.; George, F.M.; Neves, F.D.D.; Mendonca, G. Influence of operator experience, scanner type, and scan size on 3D scans. *J. Prosthet. Dent.* **2021**, *125*, 294–299. [CrossRef]
33. Lawson, N.C.; Burgess, J.O.; Litaker, M. Tear strength of five elastomeric impression materials at two setting times and two tearing rates. *J. Esthet. Restor. Dent.* **2008**, *20*, 186–193. [CrossRef]
34. Schubert, O.; Erdelt, K.J.; Tittenhofer, R.; Hajto, J.; Bergmann, A.; Guth, J.F. Influence of intraoral scanning on the quality of preparations for all-ceramic single crowns. *Clin. Oral Investig.* **2020**, *24*, 4511–4518. [CrossRef]
35. Park, S.; Kang, H.C.; Lee, J.; Shin, J.; Shin, Y.G. An enhanced method for registration of dental surfaces partially scanned by a 3D dental laser scanning. *Comput. Methods Programs Biomed.* **2015**, *118*, 11–22. [CrossRef] [PubMed]
36. Walker, M.P.; Alderman, N.; Petrie, C.S.; Melander, J.; McGuire, J. Correlation of impression removal force with elastomeric impression material rigidity and hardness. *J. Prosthodont.* **2013**, *22*, 362–366. [CrossRef] [PubMed]

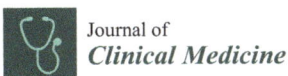

Article

Accuracy of DICOM–DICOM vs. DICOM–STL Protocols in Computer-Guided Surgery: A Human Clinical Study

Gianmaria D'Addazio [1,2], Edit Xhajanka [3], Tonino Traini [1,2], Manlio Santilli [1,2], Imena Rexhepi [1,2], Giovanna Murmura [1], Sergio Caputi [1,2] and Bruna Sinjari [1,2,*]

1. Unit of Prosthodontics, Department of Innovative Technologies in Medicine and Dentistry, University "G. d'Annunzio" Chieti-Pescara, 66100 Chieti, Italy; gianmariad@gmail.com (G.D.); t.traini@unich.it (T.T.); santilliman@gmail.com (M.S.); imena.rexhepi@unich.it (I.R.); giovanna.murmura@unich.it (G.M.); scaputi@unich.it (S.C.)
2. Electron Microscopy Laboratory, University "G. d'Annunzio" Chieti-Pescara, 66100 Chieti, Italy
3. Department of Dental Medicine, Medical University of Tirana, Rruga e Dibrës, 1001 Tirana, Albania; editxhajanka@yahoo.com
* Correspondence: b.sinjari@unich.it; Tel.: +39-392-27471479; Fax: +39-0871-3554070

Abstract: Guided implant surgery can enhance implant placement positioning, increasing predictability and decreasing postoperative complications., To date, the best protocol to be used for template realization is still unknown. Thus, the aim herein was to clinically compare the accuracy of two different protocols. A total of 48 implants were divided into Group A (24 implants), in which a stereolithographic template was realized using the digital imaging and communications in medicine (DICOM) data arrived from cone beam computer tomographies (CBCTs) (patients and prothesis alone), and Group B (24 implant), in which a standard intraoral stent with a standardized extraoral support was used for patients' intraoral impressions and CBCT. The preimplant virtual planning and postsurgery CBCT images of both groups were superimposed, and differences were registered in terms of average deviations at the platform (a) and implant apex (b), mean depth change (c), and angular deviation (d). The results demonstrated that there were no statistically significant differences between groups ($p = 0.76$) for the parameters measured. However, statistically significant differences ($p < 0.05$) were found between maxillary and mandible implant surgery, as the latter showed greater accuracy. Additional studies are necessary to further reduce discrepancies between planning and surgical procedures.

Keywords: dental implants; guided surgery; digital workflow; stereolithographic surgical guide; accuracy; CAD–CAM; DICOM–STL; static guided surgery

1. Introduction

To date, the use of implants in totally edentulous patients or patients with residual dentition has allowed for safe and predictable patient rehabilitation [1,2]. Over the years, different solutions have been developed, depending on the degree of atrophy and patients' needs [3–5]. The success of rehabilitations depends on various factors, such as appropriate presence of hard and soft tissues, healthy systematic conditions, macro- and microimplant morphologies, correct positioning, and maintenance over the years [6–12]. The use of computer-guided surgery has made it possible to simplify procedures and carry out guided prosthetic rehabilitation, also allowing immediate loading procedures [13–15]. In this sense, computer-guided surgery represents a valid method for treating patients with extensive rehabilitations [13–15]. Through detailed planning, this ensures correct three-dimensional positioning while respecting the residual bone and prosthetic position [14–17]. Several studies and literature reviews have investigated the advantages and limitations of computer-guided surgery [18–21]. The advantages include the possibility of reducing trauma and the duration of surgical interventions, avoiding errors and complications [14–16,22]. On the other hand, any design errors in the size of the template, and consequently the impossibility of deviating from the initial design, can fall within the limits of computer-guided static surgery [16,21,23–26]. However, errors during the various steps can cause different positioning than was planned, thus eliminating the advantages of computer-guided implant insertion. These errors are mainly attributable to mistakes made during data collection, planning, or the creation of surgical templates [18–21,24] Even if the growth of dental digital technologies has significantly reduced the errors in terms of angular deviation, apex or coronal portion of the implant, and insertion depth, minimal differences between the planned and real position of the implants till remain [21]. In this regard, cone beam computerized tomography (CBCT) and intra- or extraoral scanning play key roles [27,28]. CBCT is useful for the visualization of hard tissues [27], while intra- and extraoral scanning allow obtaining information on soft tissues and prostheses [17]. Overlaying the aforementioned collected data creates a virtual patient that can be used for implant planning procedures [13,22]. Through this workflow, it is possible to obtain resin guides for implant positioning through different production processes such as milling, rapid prototyping, stereolithography, and 3D printing [29]. However, the working protocols for the aforementioned data collection are different. In fact, it is the data collection, among other steps, that can cause discrepancies by increasing the possibility of error [30–32]. To date, three systems have been described for the collection and matching of patients' data that allow, through different procedures, the overlapping of information from hard tissues (both bone and teeth) and soft tissues for prosthetic planning. These three systems are: DICOM–cast, DICOM–DICOM, and DICOM–STL (standard triangulation language) [30–32]. In the DICOM–cast system, a radiographic template with radiopaque markers is made from a plaster model of the patient. The cast is calibrated on a parallelometer to know exactly where the reference points were inserted. Through this technique, the surgical template is always constructed from the model to have total correspondence between the position chosen for the implants and the positions determined for the radiopaque reference points [31].

The DICOM–DICOM protocol, or double-scan protocol, has been widely documented in the literature and is among the most widely used methods [30]. In this case, a radiographic template (with radiopaque marks) is used to obtain two sets of DICOM data. The first is obtained from CBCT performed on the patient with the radiographic template inserted. The second ones are obtained from CBCT performed on the radiographic template only (without the patient). The two sets of data are then overlaid through the common points (radiopaque marks) in both sets of data [30].

The DICOM–STL protocol is based on overlapping between the DICOM data obtained from the patient's CBCT and the STL data obtained from an impression (intra- or extraoral cast scanning) [32]. Common points, understood as areas visible on both the DICOM and the STL file, are used to superimpose the two sets of data. They are represented by the teeth in case of partially edentulous patients and by an extraoral stent linked with the patient's prosthesis in the case of totally edentulous patients. Extraoral stents are radiopaque and thus visible on DICOM images. Moreover, they present a shape that can be detected by the scanner (for the STL image). For this technique, extraoral reference points of known geometric shape could be matched between CBCT and STL file [32].

Several studies have compared the actual position of the inserted implants with the planned position to understand the accuracy of the digital techniques [33]. However, to the best of the authors' knowledge, no study has ever analyzed data coupling techniques to determine which has the greatest sensitivity and smallest margin of error during surgery. Therefore, the aim of this in vivo study was to investigate the clinical accuracy of two different protocols for data matching and the realization of surgical templates, specifically DICOM–DICOM vs. DICOM–STL. The null hypothesis was that there were no differences between the two protocols in terms of precision and accuracy.

2. Materials and Methods

2.1. Study Design

For this study, 10 patients were recruited, 5 per group. A total of 48 implants were inserted. Recruited patients were 7 men and 3 women, aged between 48 and 92 years. All patients were selected according to the inclusion and exclusion criteria presented below. None of the patients was a smoker. All patients underwent preliminary CBCT examination to establish the possibility of implant insertion.

Inclusion criteria for the present study were:

1. patients of both binary genders and all races, aged between 18 and 99 years;
2. patients for whom full supportive implant rehabilitation with multiple implants was already established;
3. patients physically able to tolerate surgical and prosthetic procedures;
4. patients who agreed to going back to the dental clinic for a follow-up visit.

The exclusion criteria were:

1. patients with active infection or severe inflammation in the areas identified for implant placement;
2. patients with a smoking habit exceeding 10 cigarettes per day;
3. patients with uncontrolled diabetes or metabolic bone disease or other uncontrolled systemic diseases;
4. patients with a history of radiotherapy treatment of the craniofacial area;
5. patients with a known gestational state;
6. patients with evidence of severe bruxism or grinding;
7. patients requiring augmentation procedures for dental implant placement and/or with buccal–lingual bone ridge dimensions of less than 5 mm.

All patients were rehabilitated with full implant supported rehabilitations performed by computer guided surgery. For all patients, data were collected, and surgical guides were constructed, according to the company's instructions. Specifically, patients were randomly divided into two groups:

Group A: Five patients treated with mucosa-supported surgical guides made using the DICOM–DICOM protocol (or double scan protocol) (Nobel Biocare Services AG P.O. Box CH-8058 Zurich-Flughafen Switzerland).

Group B: Five patients treated with mucosa-supported surgical guides made using the DICOM–STL protocol (or extraoral stent protocol) (GEASS srl Via Madonna della Salute, 23 33050 Pozzuolo del Friuli, UD).

Data collection, template production, and clinical phases are described below. Following the indications of the producers, the data were collected in different ways. Specific surgical guides were produced for each patient with dedicated components according to the group they belonged to. Patients from both groups were rehabilitated with 4 or 6 implants depending on individual diagnostic evaluations. Specifically, each group included 2 complete rehabilitations on 6 implants and 3 complete rehabilitations on 4 implants for a total of 48 implants (24 per group).

In order to reduce the variables of the study, all interventions were performed by the same surgeon, changing only the data collection protocol and consequently the template production and implant type. In cases in which the insertion torque was greater than 35 Ncm, the implant was used for immediate loading rehabilitation [34].

2.2. Data Acquisition and Templates Realization

Both protocols involved the fabrication of a denture or a duplicate of the patient's own denture in radiopaque resin.

Briefly, in Group A, as prescribed by the company guidelines, the gutta-percha markers (on the vestibular and palatal–lingual sides) were inserted into 1 mm deep niches on the prosthesis. Then, the prosthesis was stabilized in the patient's mouth; the patient underwent

CBCT scanning while wearing the denture, and subsequently, CBCT of the denture alone was performed. Images from the two different protocols are shown in Figure 1.

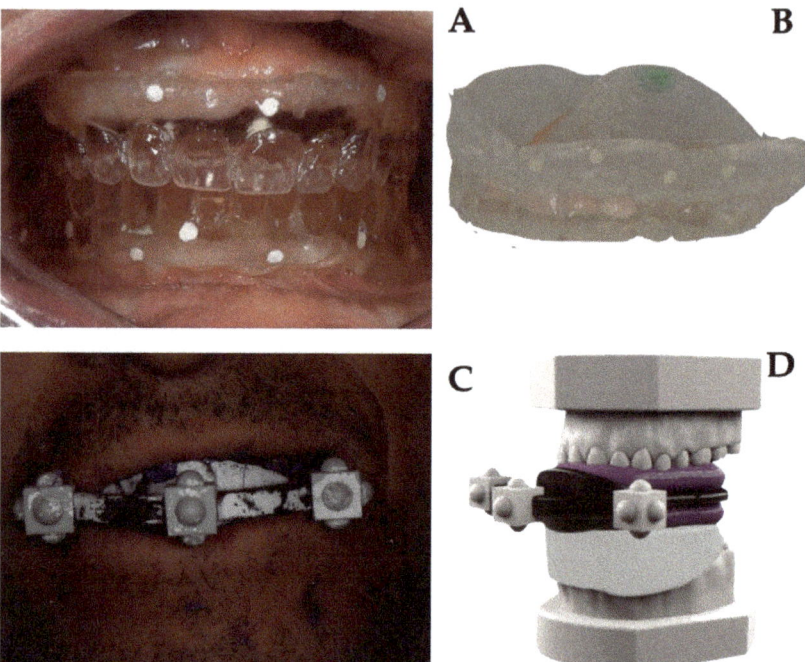

Figure 1. Data acquisition protocol: (**A**) intraoral position of resin duplicates of patient's prosthesis. Gutta-percha markers were inserted into 1 mm deep niches on the prosthesis (on the vestibular and palatal–lingual sides). The patient underwent CBCT (Cone Beam Computed Tomography) scanning while wearing the denture; (**B**) a second CBCT of the denture alone was performed; (**C**) a duplicate of the prosthesis was attached to an extraoral stent with three-dimensional radiopaque marks. The whole was stabilized in the mouth with a radiolucent occlusal index. The patient underwent CBCT scanning while wearing the duplicate, stent, and stabilization index; (**D**) extraoral scans were performed using a laboratory scanner of all collected data.

The obtained two sets of DICOM files were imported into the guided surgery software, through which the exact positions of the implants and the stabilization pins were planned in accordance with the anatomy and position of the patients' teeth. Then, the planning data were sent to produce the stereolithographic templates.

In Group B, the duplicate of the prosthesis was attached to an extraoral stent with three-dimensional radiopaque marks and then stabilized in the mouth with a radiolucent occlusal index. The patient underwent CBCT scanning while wearing the duplicate, stent, and stabilization index. Subsequently, the following scans were performed in the dental laboratory by using a laboratory scanner (Sirona InEos X5, Dentsply Sirona Italia, Piazza dell'Indipendenza, 11, 00185 Roma RM, Italy):

- master model with radiological template and stent;
- master model at the mucosal level;
- master model without stent with only radiological template in place;
- opposite arch model.

Details of data acquisition are shown in Figure 1.

The files obtained, specifically DICOM and STL files, were imported into the guided surgery software and coupled to trace more visible landmarks. The implants were then designed in terms of length, diameter, depth, vestibulobuccal inclination, and mesiodistal inclination. After the planning phase, the template file was printed by using 3D printing (Ackuretta freeshape 120, Ackuretta technologies, 11493, Taiwan, Taipei City, Neihu District, Section 1, Neihu Rd, 322 6F).

2.3. Surgical Phase

All surgeries were performed by a single operator (G.D.) Prior to surgery, the surgical guide was tested on the model and in the patient's mouth to verify correct positioning and stability. If an adequate width of keratinized gingival tissue was available at the implant site, a flapless approach was chosen; otherwise, an open-flap surgery was performed. Local anesthesia was then administered (4% articaine with adrenaline 1:100,000). The surgical guide was positioned and anchored by three bicortical bone pins. After fixation of the template, the implant sites were prepared according to the protocols provided by the manufacturers in the different groups. All drills had physical stops at the top of the drill to allow depth control. Following the standard protocol of the surgical guide system, guided milling procedures were performed, and the fixtures were inserted into the implant through the surgical guide sleeve (fully guided insertion).

Specifically, the surgical guide was fixed in the patient's mouth by fixation pins positioned buccally. The drills were passed through the metal sleeves in sequence. Once the length and diameter predetermined by the planning were reached, the implants were inserted by using a specific mounter for guided surgery that allowed for guided insertion of the implant until the desired position was reached. In the case of surgery with a flap, a suture with simple detached stitches was placed. In all cases, oral antibiotic therapy, anti-inflammatory therapy, and mouth rinses with chlorhexidine 0.20% for 7 days were prescribed.

2.4. Prosthetic Phase

All patients were rehabilitated with immediate loading fixed prostheses. Implants that did not reach a minimum insertion torque were excluded from immediate loading as previously explained [34]. The provisional prostheses were made thanks to the CAD project before implant insertion. On the surgery day, they were relined and solidified to the implant abutments. Specifically, MUAs (multiunit abutments) were placed on the implants and never removed again. Over these, temporary abutments were used for immediate loading and subsequently replaced with definitive abutments linked to the definitive prosthesis in the laboratory. The cases were finalized six months after immediate loading. Depending on the project, restorations were made in zirconia or in reinforced resin.

2.5. Data Analysis

A control CBCT was used to verify correct positioning of the implants. The same CBCT was used to verify discrepancies between the virtual plan and the actual implant position. The planning images and postoperative CBCT radiological images were overlaid by using the software's registration algorithm aimed to verify the actual position compared with the virtual planning on the same dataset. Dataset was exported in STL format, and using the software's best-fit algorithm, the image of the implant was then isolated and coupled with the corresponding implant project file to measure the deviation between the positions (Geomagic, Geomagic, Morrisville, NC, USA).

The following positional and angular deviations were calculated (as shown in Figure 2):

- A: deviation at the implant platform as the spatial distance between the center of the platform of the planned and positioned implants;
- B: deviation of the implant apex as the deviation at the apex level of the planned implant;
- C: implant depth deviation as the distance of the planned and positioned implants on the vertical axis;
- D: implant angular deviation the spatial angle between the planned and the positioned.

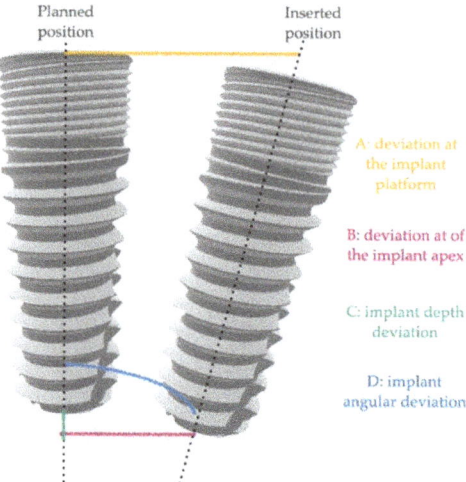

Figure 2. Graphical representation of the measurements. Differences between planned and inserted position were registered as: A—deviation at the implant platform, B—deviation of the implant apex, C—implant depth deviation, and D—implant angular deviation.

All measurements were repeated three times by two blinded researchers to verify the reproducibility of the record performed. Images from data analysis as shown in Figure 3.

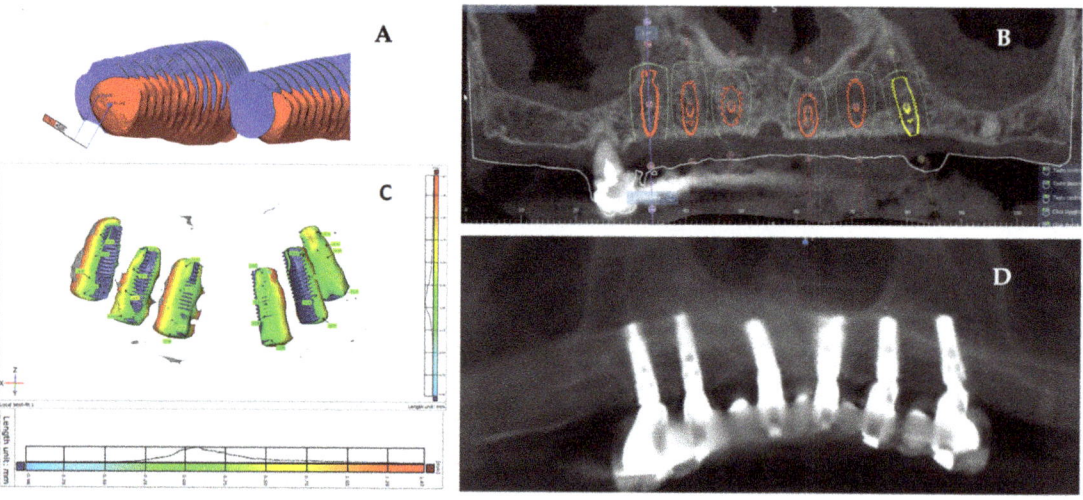

Figure 3. Data analysis: (**A**,**C**) superimposition of implant planning and postoperative CBCT images. It is possible to graphically see the discrepancy between the inserted and planned implants; (**B**,**D**) preoperative CBCT images with virtually inserted implants used for fabrication of surgical template; image of the postintervention control CBCT.

2.6. Statistical Analysis

According to Vieira et al. 2013 [16], a sample size of 21 implants per group was calculated to have at the follow-up a minimum difference between the two groups. Vieira et al. reported means of 2.17 ± 0.87 and 1.42 ± 0.76 in the two groups. The value of α was determined at 0.05, while the power of the test was 0.80. The website https://clincalc.

com/stats/samplesize.aspx (accessed on 3 July 2021) was used for the calculation [35]. A sample size increase by 10% was calculated to avoid patient losses at follow-up, which would invalidate the test. Therefore, 24 implants per group were selected.

Data were collected on different patients treated with different protocols to evaluate the differences between the two groups in terms of positional discrepancy. All data collected were processed with the same methodology to unify the results collected. The variables of interest were deviation at the implant platform, deviation at the apex of the implant, depth deviation, and angular deviation. Mean value, standard deviation, and range were used to describe the quantitative data. Data were analyzed with descriptive statistics to assess whether they had a normal distribution. The two-sample t-test and the ANOVA test (analysis of variance) were used to examine differences between the groups. Tukey tests were used to evaluate the overall significance and to perform all pairwise comparisons of the measurements between individual rehabilitation. Data analysis was performed using GraphPad version 8 statistical software. The significance level was set at $p = 0.05$.

2.7. Ethical Consideration

Participants received an information sheet and provided their informed consent in accordance with the EU General Data Protection Regulation GDPR (UE) n. 2016/679 before beginning the rehabilitation. The study protocol was postapproved by the Ethical Committee of the University of Medicine of Tirana on 3 November 2021. The allocation between groups was performed randomly. Additionally, patients were informed of the nature of the study and decided to freely take part in it.

3. Results

A total of 48 implants were placed in 10 edentulous patients. Specifically, in Group A, 16 implants were placed in the mandible and 8 in the maxilla, while in Group B, 10 implants were placed in the maxilla and 14 in the mandible. Table 1 shows the main characteristics of the patients and the inserted implants. Six patients were rehabilitated with full arches supported by four implants and four with arches supported by six implants, depending on prosthetic design and bone availability. Six months after implant placement, all included patients underwent follow-up visits to assess osseointegration before proceeding with the final prosthesis. No biological and mechanical complications were recorded. Moreover, at the one-year follow up, no intraoperative complications or implant failures were recorded, demonstrating a 100% survival rate. Table 1 shows the complications encountered during the entire study. In all rehabilitations, margins of error between the implant placed and the presurgical project were registered. However, no complications related to the placement or use of the surgical guide were observed during surgery. For all 48 implants placed, the mean deviation at the implant platform (A) was 0.803 ± 0.433 mm, while that at the apex of the implant (B) was 1.20 ± 0.484 mm. The mean change in depth (C) was 1.22 ± 0.65 mm, and the mean angular deviation (D) was $4.186 \pm 1.486°$. There were no statistically significant differences between the two groups $p = 0.76$ (A); $p = 0.35$ (B); $p = 0.81$ (C); $p = 0.62$ (D), accepting the null hypothesis. Tables 2 and 3 show all differences recorded between planned and inserted implants. Figure 4 shows statistical analysis and differences between groups. Subsequently, Tukey multiple comparisons were made between individual patients. In this case, statistically significant differences ($p < 0.05$) were found between some rehabilitations. Specifically, maxillary and mandibular rehabilitations showed major differences, as mandibular restoration showed greater precision, as demonstrated in Table 4 and Figure 5. Finally, Figure 6 and Video S1 (added as Supplementary Materials) show two different clinical cases for better understanding of the study.

Table 1. The table shows the main data of the treated patients. It also shows the main complications during surgical and prosthetic stages.

Patient ID	Sex	Age	Group	Implant Site	Final Torque	Immediate Loading	Six Month Complication	One Year Complication
1	M	48	A	47	45	Yes	No complication recorded	Screw loosening on one abutment. It was retightened at 15 Ncm
				46	55	Yes		
				44	60	Yes		
				34	50	Yes		
				36	35	No		
				37	55	Yes		
2	M	64	A	46	40	Yes	Screw loosening on one abutment. It was retightened at 15 Ncm	Bleeding on implants 46 and 36. Patient needed oral hygiene and instructions
				44	45	Yes		
				43	30	No		
				32	45	Yes		
				34	40	Yes		
				36	60	Yes		
3	M	64	A	14	40	Yes	No complication recorded	Occlusal adjustment
				12	50	Yes		
				22	55	Yes		
				24	40	Yes		
4	M	68	A	46	65	Yes	No complication recorded	No complication recorded
				32	55	Yes		
				34	50	Yes		
				36	55	Yes		
5	F	57	A	14	40	Yes	No complication recorded	No complication recorded
				12	30	No		
				22	55	Yes		
				24	45	Yes		
6	F	83	B	12	45	Yes	No complication recorded	Screw loosening on one abutment. It was retightened at 15 Ncm
				22	50	Yes		
				24	45	Yes		
				25	45	Yes		
7	M	92	B	44	45	Yes	No complication recorded	No complication recorded
				42	40	Yes		
				32	40	Yes		
				34	50	Yes		
8	M	69	B	16	50	Yes	Fracture of the prosthesis with immediate loading in the portion where there was a tooth in extension [26]	No complication recorded
				14	45	Yes		
				12	30	No		
				22	30	No		
				24	45	Yes		
				25	45	Yes		

Table 1. Cont.

Patient ID	Sex	Age	Group	Implant Site	Final Torque	Immediate Loading	Six Month Complication	One Year Complication
9	M	69	B	46	60	Yes	Screw loosening on two abutments. They were retightened at 15 Ncm	Relining was necessary to improve the fit between the prosthesis and the gingiva
				44	55	Yes		
				43	30	No		
				32	45	Yes		
				34	50	Yes		
				36	50	Yes		
10	F	73	B	44	55	Yes	No complication recorded	No complication recorded
				42	45	Yes		
				34	50	Yes		
				32	45	Yes		

Table 2. Deviation measured in patients of group A.

Patient ID	Implant Position	Deviation at the Implant Platform (A)	Deviation at the Implant Apex (B)	Implant Depth Deviation (C)	Implant Angular Deviation (D)
1 (A)	47	1.22	1.5	1.09	3.39
	46	0.45	0.98	1.12	4.15
	44	0.32	0.48	0.98	3.87
	34	0.6	1.01	1.32	6.32
	36	0.35	1.45	0.45	5.09
	37	1.12	1.32	0.76	3.76
2 (A)	46	0.98	1.17	0.23	3.12
	44	0.43	0.49	1.23	4.54
	43	0.66	0.98	2.09	5.98
	32	0.54	0.74	1.45	6.09
	34	0.76	1.09	0.79	0.98
	36	0.32	0.99	0.99	1.23
3 (A)	14	1.43	2.34	1.34	6.96
	12	1.13	1.54	1.98	4.56
	22	1.42	1.87	2.09	5.78
	24	1.8	1.95	2.45	7.09
4 (A)	46	0.25	0.34	3.09	2.87
	32	0.54	0.65	1.12	4.56
	34	0.39	0.51	0.43	3.09
	36	0.5	0.61	1.67	3.54
5 (A)	14	1.01	1.23	0.21	3.89
	12	1.22	1.48	0.12	2.62
	22	1.48	1.54	0.43	1.32
	24	0.78	1.01	1.36	2.85
Mean		0.8208 mm	1.1362 mm	1.1995 mm	4.0687°
St. Dev		0.4449 mm	0.5114 mm	0.7514 mm	1.7184°

Table 3. Deviation measured in patients of group B.

Patient ID	Implant Position	Deviation at the Implant Platform	Deviation at the Implant Apex	Implant Depth Deviation	Implant Angular Deviation
6 (B)	12	1.34	1.43	1.21	3.56
	22	1.61	1.92	1.08	3.47
	24	1.87	1.97	0.45	5.67
	25	0.82	1.76	0.67	4.21
7 (B)	44	0.34	0.87	0.95	4.78
	42	0.41	0.93	1.31	6.09
	32	0.76	1.04	0.43	5.82
	34	0.56	0.93	1.93	5.09
8 (B)	16	0.76	0.93	0.65	3.86
	14	0.92	1.04	1.43	4.15
	12	0.32	0.43	1.37	3.98
	22	0.4	0.57	0.65	5.12
	24	0.78	1.03	0.39	4.82
	25	1.25	1.43	2.09	2.12
9 (B)	46	1.12	1.78	2.12	3.06
	44	1.09	2.09	1.87	3.87
	43	0.72	1.68	0.82	3.1
	32	0.1	0.67	1.45	3.06
	34	0.34	1.54	1.98	2.08
	36	0.65	1.45	1.65	3.95
10 (B)	44	0.45	0.87	1.38	4.02
	42	0.98	1.41	1.95	4.51
	34	0.7	1.23	1.12	5.91
	32	0.58	1.37	0.86	7.01
Mean		0.7862 mm	1.2654 mm	1.2420 mm	4.3045°
St. Dev		0.4299 mm	0.4580 mm	0.5587 mm	1.2390°

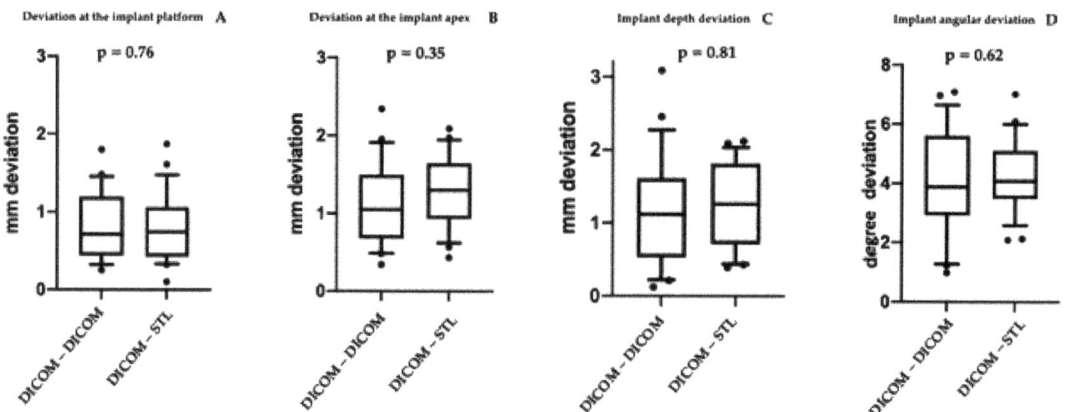

Figure 4. Images of the statistical comparisons between the two groups. The different positional and angular deviations analyzed did not show statistically significant differences.

Table 4. Tukey multiple comparisons between patients. The only significant results are reported here. In all cases, differences emerged between maxillary and mandibula rehabilitation.

Tukey's Multiple Comparisons Test	Mean Diff.	95.00% CI of Diff.	Sig.	Adjusted *p* Value
deviation at the implant platform (A)				
ID1 A vs. ID3 A	−0.7683	−1.460 to −0.07632	Yes	0.0195
ID1 A vs. ID6 B	−0.7333	−1.425 to −0.04132	Yes	0.0303
ID2 A vs. ID3 A	−0.83	−1.522 to −0.1380	Yes	0.0087
ID2 A vs. ID6 B	−0.795	−1.487 to −0.1030	Yes	0.0138
ID3 A vs. ID4 A	1.025	0.2669 to 1.783	Yes	0.002
ID3 A vs. ID7 B	0.9275	0.1694 to 1.686	Yes	0.0069
ID3 A vs. ID9 B	0.775	0.08299 to 1.467	Yes	0.0179
ID3 A vs. ID10 B	0.7675	0.009440 to 1.526	Yes	0.0451
ID4 A vs. ID6 B	−0.99	−1.748 to −0.2319	Yes	0.0032
ID6 B vs. ID7 B	0.8925	0.1344 to 1.651	Yes	0.0107
ID6 B vs. ID9 B	0.74	0.04799 to 1.432	Yes	0.0279
deviation at the implant apex (B)				
ID1 A vs. ID3 A	−0.8017	−1.485 to −0.1183	Yes	0.0111
ID2 A vs. ID3 A	−1.015	−1.698 to −0.3316	Yes	0.0005
ID2 A vs. ID6 B	−0.86	−1.543 to −0.1766	Yes	0.005
ID3 A vs. ID4 A	1.398	0.6489 to 2.146	Yes	<0.0001
ID3 A vs. ID7 B	0.9825	0.2339 to 1.731	Yes	0.003
ID4 A vs. ID5 A	−0.7875	−1.536 to −0.03890	Yes	0.0324
ID4 A vs. ID6 B	−1.243	−1.991 to −0.4939	Yes	<0.0001
ID6 B vs. ID7 B	0.8275	0.07890 to 1.576	Yes	0.0204
ID8 B vs. ID9 B	−0.63	−1.241 to −0.01877	Yes	0.0388
Implant angular deviation (D)				
ID3 A vs. ID9 B	2.911	0.2288 to 5.593	Yes	0.0243

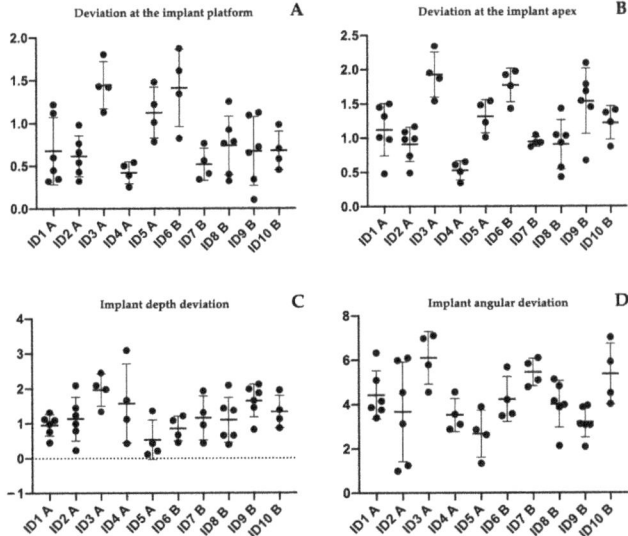

Figure 5. Images of statistical comparisons between the single treated patients. Tukey multiple comparison showed some statistically significant differences between patients. Specifically, as detailed in Table 4, statistically significant differences appeared between maxillary and mandibular rehabilitation. (**A**) Deviation at implant platform among all patients; (**B**) deviation at implant apex among all patients; (**C**) depth deviation among all patients; (**D**) angular deviation among all patients.

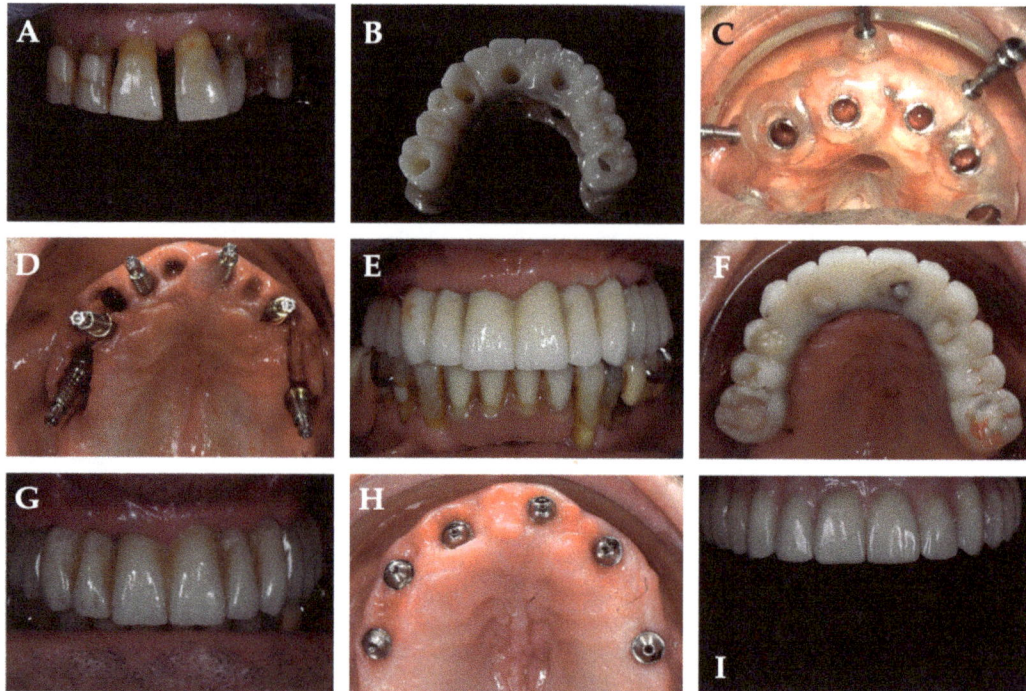

Figure 6. Demonstrative case from one of the treated patients: (**A**) preoperative image of hopeless dentition. Patient was rehabilitated with full arch supported by 6 implants; (**B**) CAD–CAM-milled temporary prosthesis in PMMA with metal palatal reinforcement. The provisional was perforated at the level of the prosthetic emergencies in order to be positioned and fixed after implant insertion; (**C**) surgical template positioned and fixed with 3 vestibular pins; (**D**) intraoral image with inserted implants and abutments; (**E**) frontal image of immediate loading provisional prosthesis; (**F**) occlusal image of immediate loading provisional prosthesis; (**G**) six-month control visit of the provisional restoration; (**H**) occlusal image of the abutments and soft tissues six months after implant insertion; (**I**) definitive restoration.

4. Discussion

Over the years, the use of CAD–CAM technologies and computer-guided surgery has enabled extensive rehabilitations to be carried out, thus reducing morbidity and postoperative discomfort and improving the predictability of restorations [17,18,21]. Thanks to these technologies, it is possible to establish the exact position of the implant in relation to the residual bone and the design of the patient's prosthesis. Among other aspects, this reduces the surgery time and allows the prosthesis to be made properly before surgery [15]. This is all possible thanks to strict protocols established over the years, which have made it possible to standardize presurgical and surgical procedures [30]. Key factors, such as materials for surgical templates and presurgical planning, have been extensively studied to reduce the margins of error [16,21,33]. The aim of the presented study was to investigate the clinical accuracy of two different protocols for data matching and surgical templates realization. This aspect has been little investigated in the literature, and the aim was to establish which was the best protocol.

The results showed that in all placed implants, there was a margin of error between the planned and inserted implants. However, there were no statistically significant differences between the two groups. In this case, the null hypothesis of the study was accepted. Several studies have investigated the accuracy of computer-guided surgery by studying the discrepancy between implant planning and the surgical phase [18,33,36,37]. To date, in all cases, there have been differences, albeit minimal, between the planned position and surgery. A meta-analysis by Zhous et al. in 2018 [36] reported 14 in vivo studies with a mean deviation of 1.25 mm in the platform portion and an angular deviation of 4.1°. In addition, the authors reported an average deviation at the apex of 1.57 mm. The results reported herein demonstrated a reduction in the overall margins of error. This was probably related to the refinement of guided surgery protocols over the years. The same authors concluded that various factors, such as the type of template, fixation, presence/absence of residual teeth, and choice of flap can affect the level of accuracy [36]. Another review by Tahmaseb et al. in 2018 [18] reported lower margins of error, which were likely related to the inclusion of in vitro studies in the review, as the margin of error can be better controlled from the influence of factors such as mouth opening or patient reflexes that could interfere in in vivo studies [18]. Furthermore, recent studies have evaluated the accuracy of computer-guided surgery, leading to results comparable to those presented in the present study. Moreover, our results were in accordance with those of Lin et al. in 2020 [21], where an average global deviation of 0.78 mm at the implant platform and 1.28 mm at the implant apex were reported. In this case, the authors proposed a fully digital protocol, demonstrating how the margins of improvement over past years could further reduce the margin of error by exploiting the potential of digital dentistry [21].

Among the most critical factors reported in the literature, the accuracy of CBCT and possible micromovements of the mucosa-supported surgical template may have the greatest influence on planning [38]. The lack of significance in the comparison between the groups and the presence of an extremely low overall error showed that both proposed techniques, when performed rigorously, led to high performance of computer-guided surgery techniques. This translates into greater comfort for both clinician and patient. Moreover, it increases the possibility of reducing postoperative complications and shortening intervention times [15]. In the cases reported, there were no relevant complications. In two patients, the fixation screw of the prosthesis was unscrewed in the first six months. Unscrewing is one of the most common mechanical complications in implantology [39,40]. A correct tightening protocol allows reducing the occurrence of this complication [41]. Varvara et al. in 2020 demonstrated how a retightening time of 2 min led to significantly reduced preload loss [41].

In the second phase of the study, Tukey multiple comparisons were made among the individual arches treated. In this case, the results showed that the performed rehabilitations in the mandible were the most accurate. It must be remembered that the inclusion criteria allowed only patients with adequate bone availability to be considered. In this case, the factors to be taken into account to understand the various results may be the different stability of the template as well as the different bone architecture. The results presented were in accordance with the data obtained by Vieira et al. [16], which showed mean platform deviations of 2.17 mm in the maxilla and 1.42 mm in the mandible [16]. In agreement with these authors, we believe that the reduced bone density of the upper jaw can be considered the cause of the greater discrepancy with the mandibular bone. On the other hand, individual susceptibility in stabilizing surgical guidance should not be underestimated. The stop obtained from the upper jaw may reduce its movements compared with those of the mandible [16]. The use of fixation pins and intermaxillary positioning gigs make it possible to avoid this variable, leading to considering bone density as the only key element in the different result obtained between the two jaws. Vinci et al. in 2020 [33] concluded by showing a margin of error of less than 1 mm, with higher margins of error in the mandible [31]. This could be related to patient selection, which required less stringent criteria for bone availability. Ridge augmentation is necessary in case of severe atrophy [42]. Some authors described the possibility of using computer-guided surgery simultaneously with guided bone regeneration procedures to improve the predictability of the intervention or avoid such procedures [43,44]. Otherwise, bone augmentation procedures can be successfully implemented to restore volumes before guided implant insertion [42–44].

Within the limitations of this study, the results encourage the use of both investigated protocols in computer-guided surgery. On the other hand, the discrepancy found showed that several factors could affect this procedure, such as bone density due to anatomical differences. Therefore, the study could be expanded over time, considering more patients and evaluating further variables. In recent years, technologies have made it possible to drastically reduce the margin of error, and the results obtained show that this trend, compared with the literature of recent years, is definitely encouraging. The study, along with future improvement of technologies and protocols, could lead to the concrete elimination of this margin of error.

Supplementary Materials: The following are available online at https://zenodo.org/record/6273727#.Yhh_Ay9aaEc, (accessed on 21 April 2022), Video S1: Guided surgery and immediate loading restoration.

Author Contributions: Conceptualization, B.S. and S.C.; methodology, G.D. and E.X.; software, G.D., M.S. and E.X.; validation, T.T., B.S. and E.X.; formal analysis, M.S. and T.T.; investigation, E.X.; resources, S.C.; data curation, G.D., G.M. and I.R.; writing—original draft preparation, G.D. and E.X.; writing—review and editing, B.S. and T.T.; visualization, S.C. and G.M.; supervision, B.S.; project administration, B.S. and S.C.; funding acquisition, B.S. and S.C. All authors have read and agreed to the published version of the manuscript.

Funding: This research was supported by the internal found of the University of Chieti-Pescara (BS EX60% N. BS60/2019).

Institutional Review Board Statement: The study was conducted in accordance with the Declaration of Helsinki and post approved by the Ethics Committee of the University of Medicine of Tirana on 3 November 2021.

Informed Consent Statement: Informed consent was obtained from all subjects involved in the study.

Data Availability Statement: Not applicable.

Conflicts of Interest: The authors declare no conflict of interest.

References

1. Sinjari, B.; D'Addazio, G.; Traini, T.; Varvara, G.; Scarano, A.; Murmura, G.; Caputi, S. A 10-year retrospective comparative human study on screw-retained versus cemented dental implant abutments. *J. Biol. Regul. Homeost. Agents* **2019**, *33*, 787–797. [PubMed]
2. Trullenque-Eriksson, A.; Guisado-Moya, B. Retrospective long-term evaluation of dental implants in totally and partially edentulous patients. Part I: Survival and marginal bone loss. *Implant Dent.* **2014**, *23*, 732–737. [CrossRef]
3. Merli, M.; Moscatelli, M.; Pagliaro, U.; Mariotti, G.; Merli, I.; Nieri, M. Implant prosthetic rehabilitation in partially edentulous patients with bone atrophy. An umbrella review based on systematic reviews of randomised controlled trials. *Eur. J. Oral Implantol.* **2018**, *11*, 261–280. [PubMed]
4. Merlone, A.; Tetè, G.; Cantile, N.; Manacorda, M.; Cattoni, F. Minimally invasive digital implant-prosthetic procedure in "all on 4" rehabilitation in patients with special needs: A three-year follow-up. *J. Biol. Regul. Homeost. Agents* **2021**, *35*, 71–85. [PubMed]
5. Urban, I.A.; Monje, A.; Lozada, J.L.; Wang, H.L. Long-term Evaluation of Peri-implant Bone Level after Reconstruction of Severely Atrophic Edentulous Maxilla via Vertical and Horizontal Guided Bone Regeneration in Combination with Sinus Augmentation: A Case Series with 1 to 15 Years of Loading. *Clin. Implant Dent. Relat. Res.* **2017**, *19*, 46–55. [CrossRef]
6. Papi, P.; Di Murro, B.; Pranno, N.; Bisogni, V.; Saracino, V.; Letizia, C.; Polimeni, A.; Pompa, G. Prevalence of peri-implant diseases among an Italian population of patients with metabolic syndrome: A cross-sectional study. *J. Periodontol.* **2019**, *90*, 1374–1382. [CrossRef]
7. Valente, F.; Scarano, A.; Murmura, G.; Varvara, G.; Sinjari, B.; Mandelli, F.; Piattelli, M.; Caputi, S.; Traini, T. Collagen Fibres Orientation in the Bone Matrix around Dental Implants: Does the Implant's Thread Design Play a Role? *Int. J. Mol. Sci.* **2021**, *22*, 7860. [CrossRef]
8. Testori, T.; Weinstein, T.; Scutellà, F.; Wang, H.L.; Zucchelli, G. Implant placement in the esthetic area: Criteria for positioning single and multiple implants. *Periodontol. 2000* **2018**, *77*, 176–196. [CrossRef]
9. Malchiodi, L.; Giacomazzi, E.; Cucchi, A.; Ricciotti, G.; Caricasulo, R.; Bertossi, D.; Gherlone, E. Relationship Between Crestal Bone Levels and Crown-to-Implant Ratio of Ultra-Short Implants with a Micro-rough Surface: A Prospective Study With 48 Months of Follow-Up. *J. Oral Implantol.* **2019**, *45*, 18–28. [CrossRef]

10. Sinjari, B.; D'Addazio, G.; De Tullio, I.; Traini, T.; Caputi, S. Peri-Implant Bone Resorption during Healing Abutment Placement: The Effect of a 0.20% Chlorhexidine Gel vs. Placebo-A Randomized Double Blind Controlled Human Study. *BioMed Res. Int.* **2018**, *2018*, 5326340. [CrossRef]
11. Mangano, C.; Mangano, F.G.; Shibli, J.A.; Roth, L.A.; d'Addazio, G.; Piattelli, A.; Iezzi, G. Immunohistochemical Evaluation of Peri-Implant Soft Tissues around Machined and Direct Metal Laser Sintered (DMLS) Healing Abutments in Humans. *Int. J. Environ. Res. Public Health* **2018**, *15*, 1611. [CrossRef] [PubMed]
12. Zukauskas, S.; Puisys, A.; Andrijauskas, P.; Zaleckas, L.; Vindasiute-Narbute, E.; Linkevičius, T. Influence of Implant Placement Depth and Soft Tissue Thickness on Crestal Bone Stability Around Implants With and Without Platform Switching: A Comparative Clinical Trial. *Int. J. Periodontics Restor. Dent.* **2021**, *41*, 347–355. [CrossRef] [PubMed]
13. Venezia, P.; Torsello, F.; Santomauro, V.; Dibello, V.; Cavalcanti, R. Full Digital Workflow for the Treatment of an Edentulous Patient with Guided Surgery, Immediate Loading, and 3D-Printed Hybrid Prosthesis: The BARI Technique 2.0. A Case Report. *Int. J. Environ. Res. Public Health* **2019**, *16*, 5160. [CrossRef] [PubMed]
14. Cattoni, F.; Chirico, L.; Cantile, N.; Merlone, A. Traditional prosthetic workflow for implant rehabilitations with a reduced number of fixtures: Proposal of a protocol. *J. Biol. Regul. Homeost. Agents* **2021**, *35*, 31–40. [PubMed]
15. Makarov, N.; Pompa, G.; Papi, P. Computer-assisted implant placement and full-arch immediate loading with digitally prefabricated provisional prostheses without cast: A prospective pilot cohort study. *Int. J. Implant Dent.* **2021**, *7*, 80. [CrossRef]
16. Vieira, D.M.; Sotto-Maior, B.S.; Barros, C.A.; Reis, E.S.; Francischone, C.E. Clinical accuracy of flapless computer-guided surgery for implant placement in edentulous arches. *Int. J. Oral Maxillofac. Implant.* **2013**, *28*, 1347–1351. [CrossRef] [PubMed]
17. Wismeijer, D.; Joda, T.; Flügge, T.; Fokas, G.; Tahmaseb, A.; Bechelli, D.; Bohner, L.; Bornstein, M.; Burgoyne, A.; Caram, S.; et al. Group 5 ITI Consensus Report: Digital technologies. *Clin. Oral Implant. Res.* **2018**, *29*, 436–442. [CrossRef]
18. Tahmaseb, A.; Wu, V.; Wismeijer, D.; Coucke, W.; Evans, C. The accuracy of static computer-aided implant surgery: A systematic review and meta-analysis. *Clin. Oral Implant. Res.* **2018**, *29*, 416–435. [CrossRef]
19. Wegmüller, L.; Halbeisen, F.; Sharma, N.; Kühl, S.; Thieringer, F.M. Consumer vs. High-End 3D Printers for Guided Implant Surgery-An In Vitro Accuracy Assessment Study of Different 3D Printing Technologies. *J. Clin. Med.* **2021**, *10*, 4894. [CrossRef]
20. Mistry, A.; Ucer, C.; Thompson, J.D.; Khan, R.S.; Karahmet, E.; Sher, F. 3D Guided Dental Implant Placement: Impact on Surgical Accuracy and Collateral Damage to the Inferior Alveolar Nerve. *Dent. J.* **2021**, *9*, 99. [CrossRef]
21. Lin, C.C.; Wu, C.Z.; Huang, M.S.; Huang, C.F.; Cheng, H.C.; Wang, D.P. Fully Digital Workflow for Planning Static Guided Implant Surgery: A Prospective Accuracy Study. *J. Clin. Med.* **2020**, *9*, 980. [CrossRef] [PubMed]
22. Cattoni, F.; Chirico, L.; Merlone, A.; Manacorda, M.; Vinci, R.; Gherlone, E.F. Digital Smile Designed Computer-Aided Surgery versus Traditional Workflow in "All on Four" Rehabilitations: A Randomized Clinical Trial with 4-Years Follow-Up. *Int. J. Environ. Res. Public Health* **2021**, *18*, 3449. [CrossRef] [PubMed]
23. D'haese, R.; Vrombaut, T.; Hommez, G.; De Bruyn, H.; Vandeweghe, S. Accuracy of Guided Implant Surgery in the Edentulous Jaw Using Desktop 3D-Printed Mucosal Supported Guides. *J. Clin. Med.* **2021**, *10*, 391. [CrossRef] [PubMed]
24. Mozer, P.S. Accuracy and Deviation Analysis of Static and Robotic Guided Implant Surgery: A Case Study. *Int. J. Oral Maxillofac. Implant.* **2020**, *35*, e86–e90. [CrossRef]
25. Bover-Ramos, F.; Viña-Almunia, J.; Cervera-Ballester, J.; Peñarrocha-Diago, M.; García-Mira, B. Accuracy of Implant Placement with Computer-Guided Surgery: A Systematic Review and Meta-Analysis Comparing Cadaver, Clinical, and In Vitro Studies. *Int. J. Oral Maxillofac. Implant.* **2018**, *33*, 101–115. [CrossRef] [PubMed]
26. Guentsch, A.; Sukhtankar, L.; An, H.; Luepke, P.G. Precision, and trueness of implant placement with and without static surgical guides: An in vitro study. *J. Prosthet. Dent.* **2021**, *126*, 398–404. [CrossRef]
27. Guerrero, M.E.; Jacobs, R.; Loubele, M.; Schutyser, F.; Suetens, P.; Van Steenberghe, D. State-of-the-art on cone beam CT imaging for preoperative planning of implant placement. *Clin. Oral Investig.* **2006**, *10*, 1–7. [CrossRef]
28. Gargallo-Albiol, J.; Barootchi, S.; Salomó-Coll, O.; Wang, H.-L. Advantages, and disadvantages of implant navigation surgery. A systematic review. *Ann. Anat. Anat. Anz.* **2019**, *225*, 1–10. [CrossRef]
29. Chen, X.; Yuan, J.; Wang, C.; Huang, Y.; Kang, L. Modular Preoperative Planning Software for Computer- Aided Oral Implantology and the Application of a Novel Stereolithographic Template: A Pilot Study. *Clin. Implant. Dent. Relat. Res.* **2009**, *12*, 181–193.
30. Vercruyssen, M.; Jacobs, R.; Van Assche, N.; van Steenberghe, D. The use of CT scan-based planning for oral rehabilitation by means of implants and its transfer to the surgical field: A critical review on accuracy. *J. Oral Rehabil.* **2008**, *35*, 454–474. [CrossRef]
31. Modica, F.; Fava, C.; Benech, A.; Preti, G. Radiologic-prosthetic planning of the surgical phase of the treatment of edentulism by osseointegrated implants: An in vitro study. *J. Prosthet. Dent.* **1991**, *65*, 541–546. [CrossRef]
32. Kernen, F.; Kramer, J.; Wanner, L.; Wismeijer, D.; Nelson, K.; Flügge, T. A review of virtual planning software for guided implant surgery—Data import and visualization, drill guide design and manufacturing. *BMC Oral Health* **2020**, *20*, 251. [CrossRef] [PubMed]
33. Vinci, R.; Manacorda, M.; Abundo, R.; Lucchina, A.G.; Scarano, A.; Crocetta, C.; Muzio, L.L.; Gherlone, E.F.; Mastrangelo, F. Accuracy of Edentulous Computer-Aided Implant Surgery as Compared to Virtual Planning: A Retrospective Multicenter Study. *J. Clin. Med.* **2020**, *9*, 774. [CrossRef] [PubMed]

34. Felice, P.; Soardi, E.; Piattelli, M.; Pistilli, R.; Jacotti, M.; Esposito, M. Immediate non-occlusal loading of immediate post-extractive versus delayed placement of single implants in preserved sockets of the anterior maxilla: 4-month post-loading results from a pragmatic multicentre randomised controlled trial. *Eur. J. Oral Implantol.* **2011**, *4*, 329–344.
35. Sample Size Calculator. Available online: https://clincalc.com/stats/samplesize.aspx (accessed on 3 July 2021).
36. Zhou, W.; Liu, Z.; Song, L.; Kuo, C.L.; Shafer, D.M. Clinical Factors Affecting the Accuracy of Guided Implant Surgery-A Systematic Review and Meta-analysis. *J. Evid. Based Dent. Pract.* **2018**, *18*, 28–40. [CrossRef]
37. Rivara, F.; Lumetti, S.; Calciolari, E.; Toffoli, A.; Forlani, G.; Manfredi, E. Photogrammetric method to measure the discrepancy between clinical and software-designed positions of implants. *J. Prosthet. Dent.* **2016**, *115*, 703–711. [CrossRef]
38. Cattoni, F.; Merlone, A.; Broggi, R.; Manacorda, M.; Vinci, R. Computer-assisted prosthetic planning, and implant design with integrated digital bite registration: A treatment protocol. *J. Biol. Regul. Homeost. Agents* **2021**, *35*, 11–29.
39. D'Addazio, G.; Sinjari, B.; Arcuri, L.; Femminella, B.; Murmura, G.; Santilli, M.; Caputi, S. Mechanical Pull-Out Test of a New Hybrid Fixture-Abutment Connection: An In Vitro Study. *Materials* **2021**, *14*, 1555. [CrossRef]
40. Winkler, S.; Ring, K.; Ring, J.D.; Boberick, K.G. Implant screw mechanics and the settling effect: An overview. *J. Oral Implantol.* **2003**, *29*, 242–245. [CrossRef]
41. Varvara, G.; Sinjari, B.; Caputi, S.; Scarano, A.; Piattelli, M. The Relationship Between Time of Retightening and Preload Loss of Abutment Screws for Two Different Implant Designs: An In Vitro Study. *J. Oral Implantol.* **2020**, *46*, 13–17.
42. Cucchi, A.; Chierico, A.; Fontana, F.; Mazzocco, F.; Cinquegrana, C.; Belleggia, F.; Rossetti, P.; Soardi, C.M.; Todisco, M.; Luongo, R.; et al. Statements and Recommendations for Guided Bone Regeneration: Consensus Report of the Guided Bone Regeneration Symposium Held in Bologna, October 15 to 16, 2016. *Implant Dent.* **2019**, *28*, 388–399. [CrossRef] [PubMed]
43. Raabe, C.; Janner, S.F.M.; Abou-Ayash, S. Comprehensive Digital Workflow and Computer-Assisted Implant Surgery in a Patient with Reduced Crest Width. Case Report of a Split-Mouth Approach. *Swiss Dent. J.* **2021**, *131*, 437–441. [PubMed]
44. Poli, P.P.; Muktadar, A.K.; Souza, F.Á.; Maiorana, C.; Beretta, M. Computer-guided implant placement associated with computer-aided bone regeneration in the treatment of atrophied partially edentulous alveolar ridges: A proof-of-concept study. *J. Dent. Sci.* **2021**, *16*, 333–341. [CrossRef] [PubMed]

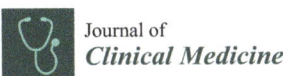

Article

Marginal Bone Maintenance and Different Prosthetic Emergence Angles: A 3-Year Retrospective Study

Diego Lops [1], Eugenio Romeo [1], Michele Stocchero [2], Antonino Palazzolo [1], Barbara Manfredi [1] and Luca Sbricoli [2,*]

[1] Department of Prosthodontics, Dental Clinic, School of Dentistry, University of Milan, 20142 Milan, Italy; diego.lops@unimi.it (D.L.); eugenio.romeo@unimi.it (E.R.); antonino.palazzolo@unimi.it (A.P.); barbara.manfredi@unimi.it (B.M.)
[2] Department of Neurosciences, School of Dentistry, University of Padova, 35128 Padova, Italy; stocchero.michele@gmail.com
* Correspondence: luca.sbricoli@unipd.it

Abstract: The aim of the present retrospective study was to assess marginal bone changes around implants restored with different prosthetic emergence profile angles. Patients were treated with implants supporting fixed dentures and were followed for 3 years. Marginal bone levels (MBL) measured at the prosthesis installation (t0) and at the 3-year follow-up visit (t1) were considered. The MBL change from t0 to t1 was investigated. Two groups were considered: Group 1 for restorations with an angle between implant axis and prosthetic emergence profile >30°, and Group 2 for those with an angle ≤30°, respectively. Moreover, peri-implant soft tissue parameters, such as the modified bleeding index (MBI) and plaque index (PI) were assessed. Seventy-four patients were included in the analysis and a total of 312 implants were examined. The mean EA in groups 1 and 2 was 45 ± 4 and 22 ± 7 degrees, respectively. The mean marginal bone level change (MBL change) of 0.06 ± 0.09 mm and 0.06 ± 0.10 mm were, respectively, in groups 1 and 2. The difference in the MBL change between the two groups was not statistically significant ($p = 0.969$). The MBL change does not seem to be influenced by the emergence angle for implants with a stable internal conical connection and platform-switching of the abutment diameter.

Keywords: dental implant; bone level; prospective study; sub-crestal placement; emergence profile

1. Introduction

Dental implants osseointegration is actually a well-established issue, due to improved surface characteristics. One of the modern implant therapy goals is to optimize esthetics, with a natural implant-supported restoration integration, especially regarding the peri-implant soft tissues. The correct interproximal papilla shape, the scalloping of the gingival margin and the thickness of the vestibular soft tissue are recognized as fundamental for esthetics. Even more important is the achievement of adequate cleansing procedures, in order to prevent any peri-implant soft tissues inflammation that may lead to a marginal bone level change. In fact, in the seventh *European Workshop on Periodontology*, different clinical parameters were recommended as items to evaluate the health status of the peri-implant tissue [1]: plaque accumulation, presence of bleeding on probing, probing depth and bone resorption, respectively.

The discrepancy between the implant diameter and the shape of the final prosthetic restoration requires compensation. According to *The Glossary of the Prosthodontic Terms*, 9th edition [2], the emergence angle (EA) is the angle between the average tangent of the transitional contour relative to the long axis of a tooth, dental implant or dental implant abutment.

Many studies have shown that over-contoured restorations may have an influence on gingival inflammation and plaque retention [3]. Excessive crown contour acts as a

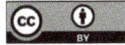

bacterial plaque accumulation factor [4], especially in the gingival third; therefore, proper oral hygiene is hindered. On the other hand, under-contoured restorations can be cleaned more easily with adequate tooth brushing techniques. In 2018, Katafuchi et al. [3] showed that an emergence angle (EA) of more than 30° is a significant risk factor for peri-implantitis and convex profiles create an additional risk for bone level implants, but not for tissue-level implants. A correlation between the restorations of EA and peri-implantitis was found in this study. Moreover, the wider the EA angle was, the greater the risk for peri-implantitis was found. Unfortunately, no data on the features of the implant to abutment connection are reported when different EAs were compared. In fact, only internal conical connection implants have proven superior to other configurations in achieving a tight seal and eliminating the microgap at the implant to abutment junction, and improvements in crestal bone maintenance [5] have been shown.

Considering the hypothesis that emergence angles of more than 30° could be a negative parameter for mid to long-term peri-implant tissues health, the aim of the present retrospective study was to analyze the influence of marginal bone level stability on restorations with different emergence angles (EA), for implants with an internal conical connection between the fixture and abutment. Moreover, how an EA angle may affect restorations in anterior or posterior areas differently, was investigated.

2. Materials and Methods

2.1. Patient Selection

Patients restored with implant fixed rehabilitation were included in the study; all cases have been treated with the same implant system (Anyridge, MegaGen Implant Co., Gyeongbuk, Korea) between 2014 and 2017; moreover, radiographic and clinical parameters taken at the time of the prosthetic delivery were assessed, so that comparisons between baseline and 3 years follow-up visit were provided.

Patients with systemic diseases, a history of radiation therapy in the head and neck region, current treatment with steroids, a neurological or psychiatric handicap that could interfere with good oral hygiene, an immuno-compromised status (including infection with human immunodeficiency virus), severe clenching or bruxism, smokers (more than 15 cigarettes per day), drug or alcohol abuse and inadequate compliance were excluded.

All included patients gave their written consent after being informed in detail about the objectives of the study. Patients with single or multiple gaps requiring fixed implant-supported restoration were included. No exclusion criteria on the edentulous site were applied. Single and multiple restorations were included.

Along with the radiograph at the time of prosthetic delivery, the following data were collected: implant diameter and length, prosthesis type, implant site position, date of prosthetic delivery. Surgical and prosthetic procedures were performed by a single operator (DL) as below described.

The STROBE (Strengthening the reporting of observational studies in epidemiology; strobe-statement.org) guidelines checklist of items was followed.

2.2. Surgical Procedures

Before treatment, patients were clinically and radiographically evaluated. Panoramic and periapical radiographs were used as a first-level exam to evaluate the bone quantity before implant placement. If a second level exam was needed to assess the alveolar ridge width, due to a suspect bone deficiency, cone beam TC was performed. For each implant, a two-stage surgical technique was chosen. Implants were placed 1 to 2 mm below the crestal level [6], as recommended by the manufacturer, according to the scalloping of the bone crest.

An inter-implant distance of 3 mm at least, and/or an interproximal space from 1.5 to 3 mm between an implant and the adjacent tooth, were observed [7–11]. A periodontal probe was used to assess the correct distances.

Flaps were sutured over the implants to allow submerged healing. If slight horizontal dehiscence was present after an implant placement, a correction by means of xenograft bone granules (Geistlich Bio-oss, Wholusen, Switzerland) was performed. A resorbable collagen membrane (Geistlich Bio-gide, Wholusen, Switzerland) was used to stabilize the graft. If requested by patients, removable prostheses or provisional fixed bridges were temporarily used during the healing period to compensate for the edentulous gaps. Surgical re-entry was performed three months later, and transmucosal healing abutments were installed.

2.3. Prosthetic Protocol

Two weeks after surgical re-entry, an implant level impression was taken for screw-retained temporary restorations. Prostheses were inserted from one to six weeks after the implant level impression. After a period of 8 to 12 weeks for peri-implant soft tissue conditioning, a definitive implant level impression was taken.

Different types of fixed restoration were selected to restore patients' edentulism: fixed single crown (SC), a partial fixed prosthesis (FPD) and full fixed prosthesis (FFD), respectively. Implants were located in the anterior jaw (central incisor to the first premolar) and in the posterior jaw (second premolar to the second molar). For cemented restorations, abutments were torqued down to 25 N/cm and restorations were cemented with temporary cement (Temp-Bond Clear, Kerr Corporation, Orange, CA, USA). On the other hand, for screw-retained prostheses, a torque of 25 N/cm was used to install the restorations by means of a proper torque wrench. After 2 weeks of loading, patients were recalled and an intraoral periapical radiograph of the restored implant site was taken; also, peri-implant clinical parameters were assessed.

2.4. Radiographic and Clinical Evaluations

All radiographs were taken with a standardized parallel technique with an X-ray apparatus supplied with a long cone and a Rinn Universal Collimator (Dentsply RINN, York, PA, USA) The following exposure parameters were used: 65–90 kV, 7.5–10 mA and 0.22–0.25 s. All radiographs were stored on a PC. Radiographic images were then analyzed with a software program (Image J, National Institute of Health, Bethesda, Rockville, MA, USA). Before measurement, each radiograph was calibrated by using the implant diameter and length as reference measures to correct any distortion.

Radiographic images were then analyzed with a software program (Image J, NIH, Montgomery County, MD, USA) to measure the following parameter: peri-implant bone level (marginal bone level, MBL). Measurements were made at the mesial and distal aspects of each implant and were reported in millimeters.

Because implants were sub-crestally positioned, measurements, where the bone crest was located coronally to the implant neck, were classified as negative values. On the contrary, measurements, where the bone crest was located apically to the implant neck, were classified as positive values.

For each implant-supported prosthesis, radiographs performed at the time of prosthetic delivery and at the follow-up visit were analyzed and compared to detect any change in the peri-implant marginal bone level. Such a procedure was carried out for each intraoral periapical radiograph by analyzing some reference measurements as: (i) implant neck diameter; (ii) implant length, by considering the distance between the implant neck and the most apical point of each implant, along an ideal line running parallel to the implant axis.

In addition, radiographs were used to measure the emergence angle (EA) between the implant long axis and the line tangent to the restoration, as described by Yotnuengnit et al. [12].

A line parallel to the implant's long axis was drawn at the outer implant neck (Figure 1). A second one was drawn tangential to the restoration from the implant to abutment connection. The angle of the intersection resulted in the emergence angle (EA). Measurements were repeated twice. Group allocation was provided by considering the definitive restoration EA angle. EA > 30° were included in Group 1 (Figure 2); conversely, EA ≤ 30° were allocated to Group 2 (Figure 3). Since implants were placed sub-crestally, the transmucosal abutment was considered a part of the restoration.

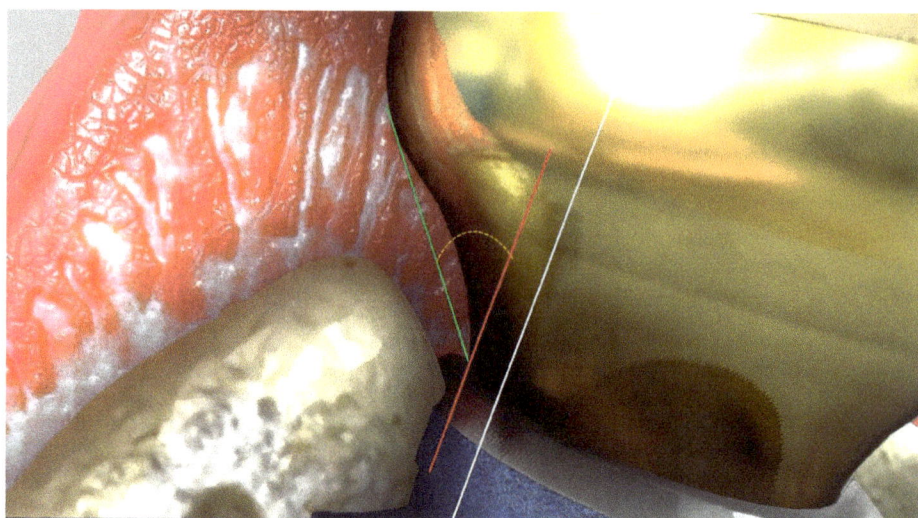

Figure 1. Emergence angle (EA) definition. White line: parallel to implant long axis. Red line: parallel to the white and tangential to the restoration from the implant to abutment connection. Green line: from implant to abutment connection point to the emergence profile. The angle of the intersection (yellow line) resulted in the emergence angle (EA).

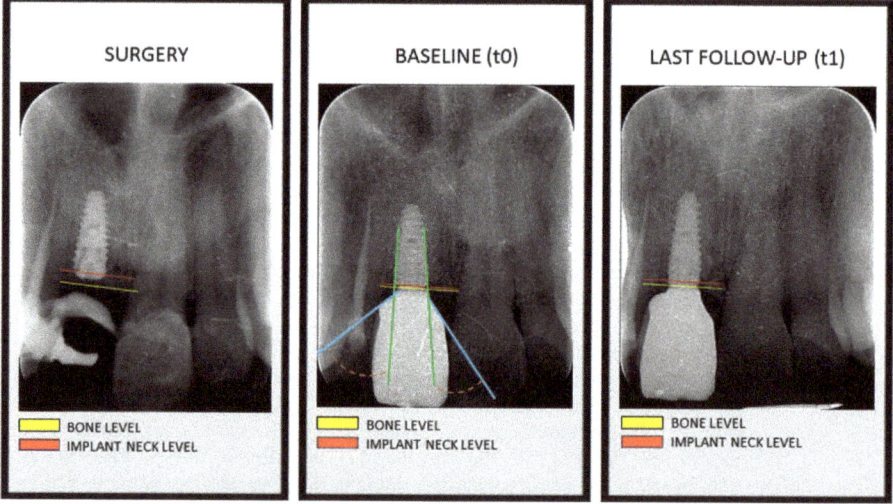

Figure 2. Bone levels at time of implant surgery, at prosthesis installation (baseline) and at last follow-up visit. Green line: implant axis. Blue line: prosthetic emergence profile axis. Orange line: angle between implant axis and prosthetic emergence profile >30°, determining the allocation in Group 1.

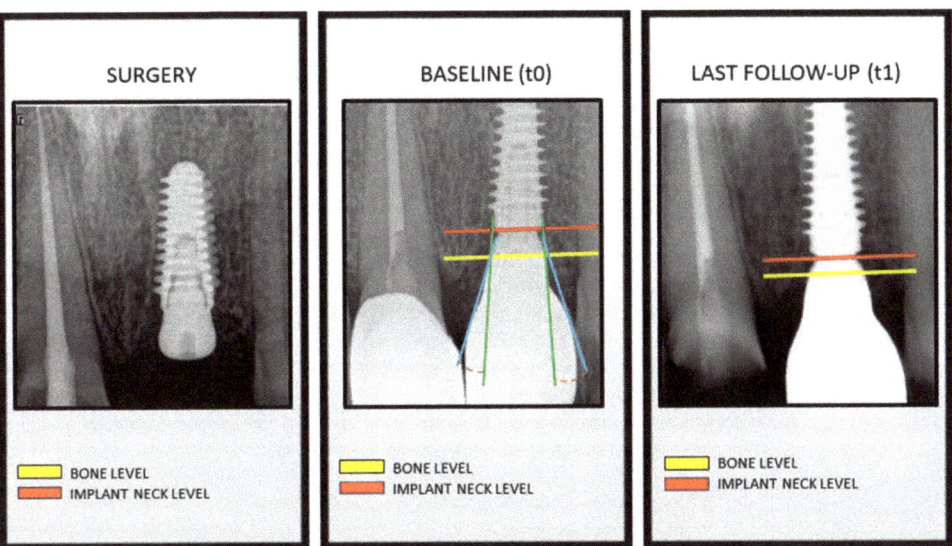

Figure 3. Bone levels at time of implant surgery, at prosthesis installation (baseline) and at last follow-up visit. Green line: implant axis. Blue line: prosthetic emergence profile axis. Orange line: angle between implant axis and prosthetic emergence profile ≤30°, determining the allocation in Group 2.

A randomization was not performed because the choice of shape and emergence angle (EA) of each prosthesis was selected by the dental technician on the specific features of the edentulous site. For both MBL and EA parameters, mean values between the mesial and distal aspects were calculated to rate the respective measurements. A single operator (MS) performed all measurements. For the emergence angle measurement, intra-operator reliability was calculated.

Additionally, peri-implant soft tissue parameters, such as the modified sulcus bleeding index (mBI) and modified plaque index (mPI) [13,14] were assessed with a calibrated plastic probe (TPS probe, Vivadent, Schaan, Liechtenstein). Both mBI and mPI scores ranged from 0 to 3. Four sites for each implant (mesial, distal, buccal and lingual) were considered for recording probing depth scores. Moreover, for mBI and mPI indexes, mean values between the mesial and distal aspects were calculated to rate the respective measurements.

2.5. Statistical Analysis

Data were collected with an implant as a unit. Descriptive statistics were performed by calculating the mean and standard deviation for continuous variables and frequency distribution for categorical variables, respectively. The distribution of the outcome was assessed by the skewness values and by a normal quartile plot. Given the hierarchical structure of the data (i.e., implants nested within patients) a preliminary linear mixed model analysis (LMM) was conducted, to estimate the between-patients variation in the outcome variable (MBL change). Therefore, a random intercepts empty model was run: only the outcome variable (i.e., MBL change) was included and the intercept (i.e., MBL change mean) was allowed. No significant variation in random intercepts, var(u0) = 0.00, $\chi^2(1) = 0.98$, $p = 0.33$ was obtained. This result showed that the outcome variable did not vary across patients and confirmed the absence of cluster effects due to the hierarchical structure of the data. Thus, a linear regression approach with MBL as the dependent variable was calculated and adopted to evaluate the role of the type of prosthesis (SC, FPD, FFD), EA (Group 1 and Group 2) and implant site (anterior vs. posterior areas).

The descriptive statistics and the model processing were developed by a statistical software package (IBM SPSS Statistics for Mac, v. 22).

3. Results

Eighty patients (38 males and 42 females, respectively) aged from 22 to 84 years (mean age 55.6 ± 32.4 years) were recruited in the present study. During the follow-up period, 6 patients (3 males and 3 females, respectively) treated with 21 implants, on the whole, did not attend the 3 years follow-up visit, so these were considered drop-outs. Only 74 patients, consecutively followed in a 3 year period from the definitive prosthesis installation, were included in the present study.

A total of 312 implants were considered and the average follow-up period was 3.8 ± 1.3 years. Implants' features of different sizes are reported in Table 1. Fixture distribution in the anterior or posterior area based on the EA type is reported in Table 2. The frequency of prosthesis type was as follows: 34 SC: single crown; 65 FPD: fixed partial denture; 12 FFD: fixed full denture. Anterior sites were considered from the first premolar to the contralateral. Conversely, implants placed in the second premolar and molar areas were included in the posterior subgroup, respectively.

Table 1. Frequency of implant length and implant diameter.

		Diameter (mm)					Total
		3.5	4	4.5	5	6.5	
	7	2	2	7	6	11	28
	8.5	4	12	1	2	9	28
Length	10	10	35	34	11	1	91
(mm)	11.5	10	6	3	1	0	20
	13	16	51	53	4	0	124
	15	17	2	2	0	0	21
Total		59	108	100	24	21	312

Table 2. Frequency of implant distribution by site of placement.

			Position		Total
			Anterior	Posterior	
Jaw	maxilla	Count	92	89	181
		% of Total	29.5%	28.5%	58.0%
	mandible	Count	45	86	131
		% of Total	14.4%	27.6%	42.0%
Total		Count	137	175	312
		% of Total	43.9%	56.1%	100.0%

The mean restorations EA in groups 1 and 2 were 45 ± 4 and 22 ± 7 degrees, respectively. EA values in Group 1 ranged from 31 to 47 degrees.

Mean marginal bone level changes (MBL change) of 0.06 ± 0.09 mm and 0.06 ± 0.10 mm were found, respectively, in groups 1 and 2 (Table 3). The MBL change in the two groups was not statistically different ($p = 0.969$). Moreover, when the MBL change of groups 1 and 2 were compared by considering the implant site (Table 3), no statistically significant difference was measured ($p = 0.611$ and 0.599, respectively, for anterior and posterior sub-groups).

Results from the linear regression for the MBL did not show a significant model using the selected parameters (type of prosthesis, EA and site location).

The mean MBI and PI values were recorded for both groups 1 and 2, respectively, at baseline and 3 years of follow-up control (Table 4).

Table 3. MBL change for different groups (Group 1: EA > 30°; Group 2: EA ≤ 30°) by implant site (anterior and posterior). N: number of implants; SD: Standard Deviation.

	Group 1		Group 2	
	N	Mean ± SD	N	Mean ± SD
Anterior	95	0.066 ± 0.09 mm	42	0.057 ± 0.11 mm
Posterior	80	0.053 ± 0.10 mm	95	0.061 ± 0.10 mm
Total	175	0.060 ± 0.09 mm	137	0.060 ± 0.10 mm

Anterior: from first premolar to the contralateral one. Posterior: second premolar and molar area.

Table 4. MBI change for different groups (Group 1: EA > 30°; Group 2: EA ≤ 30°). N: number of implants; SD: Standard Deviation.

	Group 1			Group 2		
		Baseline	Last Visit		Baseline	Last Visit
	N	Mean ± SD	Mean ± SD	N	Mean ± SD	Mean ± SD
Anterior	95	0.1 ± 0.3 mm	0.3 ± 0.2 mm	42	0.1 ± 0.2 mm	0.2 ± 0.2 mm
Posterior	80	0.3 ± 0.1 mm	0.5 ± 0.2 mm	95	0.2 ± 0.1 mm	0.4 ± 0.2 mm
Total	175	0.2 ± 0.2 mm	0.4 ± 0.3 mm	137	0.2 ± 0.2 mm	0.3 ± 0.3 mm

Anterior: from first premolar to the contralateral one. Posterior: second premolar and molar area.

The mean modified bleeding index changes (mBI change) were 0.2 and 0.1, respectively, in groups 1 and 2 (Table 3). Therefore, the mBI change in the two groups was not statistically different ($p = 0.811$). Similarly, modified plaque index changes (mPI change) were 0.2 and 0.2, respectively, in groups 1 and 2 (Table 5). Moreover, the mPI change in the two groups was not statistically different ($p = 0.365$).

Table 5. PI change for different groups (Group 1: EA > 30°; Group 2: EA ≤ 30°). N: number of implants; SD: Standard Deviation.

	Group 1			Group 2		
		Baseline	Last Visit		Baseline	Last Visit
	N	Mean ± SD	Mean ± SD	N	Mean ± SD	Mean ± SD
Anterior	95	0.0 ± 0.0 mm	0.2 ± 0.3 mm	42	0.0 ± 0.0 mm	0.2 ± 0.2 mm
Posterior	80	0.1 ± 0.1 mm	0.3 ± 0.2 mm	95	0.3 ± 0.2 mm	0.5 ± 0.3 mm
Total	175	0.05 ± 0.1 mm	0.25 ± 0.3 mm	137	0.2 ± 0.09 mm	0.4 ± 0.3 mm

4. Discussion

In the present retrospective study, the influence of the emergence angle (EA) on the marginal bone level was assessed for 312 implants placed in 74 patients after at least 3 years of function. The aim was to identify if a >30° EA might influence interproximal bone loss. The present findings partially agree with other recently published papers; a multivariate analysis to investigate the influence of prosthetic factors on the marginal bone level was conducted by Inoue et al. [15]. It was stated that there is no statistically significant correlation between the emergence angle and marginal bone level. In particular, the authors found that the marginal bone loss, after at least one year from prosthetic loading, was less for prostheses with an emergence angle between 20° and 40°. Such an outcome did not meet the present study findings, since the authors found bone stability with a mean value of 45° EA. The influence of the cervical coronal contour on marginal bone loss on 67 platform-switched implants was analyzed by Hentenaar et al. [16]. No statistically significant differences were reported between prosthetic emergence angles and marginal bone loss after 5 years of prosthetic loading. It must be recognized that only crowns with an emergence angle that did not exceed 18.7°, both on the mesial aspect and on the distal aspect, were analyzed. It is interesting, moreover, the analysis of platform-switched implants related to periodontal health parameters. The authors, in fact, found that after 5 years of prosthetic loading, the periodontal health parameters were very high, without any case of peri-implantitis. Additionally, no significant difference in both modified bleeding and plaque indices was measured at the last follow-up visit for groups 1 and 2 in the present study, respectively. Such clinical findings may show that adequate prosthetic emergence angles do not represent a risk factor for correct peri-implant soft tissues health, even if they are more than 30°.

Different results were found by Katafuchi et al. [3]. An emergence angle greater than 30° was judged to be correlated with an increased risk of peri-implantitis. However, the study by Katafuchi et al. [3] was conducted on bone-level non-platform-switched implants. Prosthetic rehabilitation on non-platform-switched bone-level implants may lead to excessively convex profiles where home hygiene maintenance is more difficult. Results comparable to those of Katafuchi were also found by Yi et al. [17]; they conducted a cross-sectional study on 349 implants 5 years after the prosthetic load in order to investigate the association between prosthetic factors and peri-implantitis. It was demonstrated that the emergence angle and emergence profile significantly affect the marginal bone level and the prevalence of peri-implantitis on bone-level implants, but not on tissue-level implants. Interestingly, the shape of the emergence profile on tissue-level implants was concave in the transmucosal part and convex in the part located above the mucosal margin.

In the present study, marginal bone loss was 0.06 mm for both EA groups after a minimum follow-up of 3 years. Such a finding agrees with previous studies [18,19] on bone stability around crestally and sub-crestally positioned implants with a platform-switching design.

The present study design suggests that the results should be interpreted with caution. One of the major drawbacks of such a clinical investigation was that the evaluation of the marginal bone level was made on the mesial and distal aspects of the implants, not taking into account the vestibular aspect. In fact, that kind of additional evaluation should require invasive 3D radiographs; for ethical reasons, such an approach was not possible to be achieved. In daily clinical practice, and particularly in the anterior area, it is now recognized that the vestibular-palatal position of the implant must be more palatal than the line that joins the center of the crowns of the adjacent teeth to allow an adequate thickness of vestibular bone [6]. This implant positioning may provide for an accentuated emergence angle if compared to the adjacent natural teeth. Another important limitation of the present study is the impossibility of controlling any confounders that could affect the stability of the marginal bone. A prospective analysis of such factors should be encouraged in the future.

5. Conclusions

Within the limits of the present investigation, with a tight and stable implant to abutment connection, an emergence angle of more than 30 degrees and less than 50 degrees may not influence the marginal bone levels' stability. Nevertheless, despite the promising outcomes on the peri-implant hard tissues stability, more prospective and long-term data are required to confirm this trend.

Author Contributions: Conceptualization, D.L. and E.R.; methodology, A.P.; investigation, B.M.; writing, L.S., D.L. and M.S.; supervision, E.R. All authors have read and agreed to the published version of the manuscript.

Funding: This research received no external funding.

Institutional Review Board Statement: The present study was conducted in accordance with the fundamental principles of the Helsinki Declaration. The Ethical Committee agreement (Prot. No. EC 02.04.20 REF 28/20) was obtained to complete the data collection procedures mentioned below.

Informed Consent Statement: Informed consent was obtained from all subjects involved in the study.

Conflicts of Interest: The authors declare no conflict of interest.

References

1. Sanz, M.; Lang, N.P.; Kinane, D.F.; Berglundh, T.; Chapple, I.; Tonetti, M.S. Seventh European Workshop on Periodontology of the European Academy of Periodontology at the Parador at La Granja, Segovia, Spain. *J. Clin. Periodontol.* **2011**, *38* (Suppl. S11), 1–2. [CrossRef] [PubMed]
2. Driscoll, C.F.; Freilich, M.A.; Guckes, A.D.; Knoernschild, K.L.; Mcgarry, T.J.; Goldstein, G.; Goodacre, C.; Guckes, A.; Mor, S.; Rosenstiel, S.; et al. The Glossary of Prosthodontic Terms: Ninth Edition. *J. Prosthet. Dent.* **2017**, *117*, e1–e105. [CrossRef]
3. Katafuchi, M.; Weinstein, B.F.; Leroux, B.G.; Chen, Y.-W.; Daubert, D.M. Restoration contour is a risk indicator for peri-implantitis: A cross-sectional radiographic analysis. *J. Clin. Periodontol.* **2018**, *45*, 225–232. [CrossRef] [PubMed]
4. Parkinson, C.F. Excessive crown contours facilitate endemic plaque niches. *J. Prosthet. Dent.* **1976**, *35*, 424–429. [CrossRef]
5. Hurson, S. Implant/Abutment Biomechanics and Material Selection for Predictable Results. *Compend. Contin. Educ. Dent.* **2018**, *39*, 440. [PubMed]
6. Lops, D.; Stocchero, M.; Jones, J.M.; Freni, A.; Palazzolo, A.; Romeo, E. Five Degree Internal Conical Connection and Marginal Bone Stability around Subcrestal Implants: A Retrospective Analysis. *Materials* **2020**, *13*, 3123. [CrossRef] [PubMed]
7. Cosyn, J.; Eghbali, A.; De Bruyn, H.; Collys, K.; Cleymaet, R.; De Rouck, T. Immediate single-tooth implants in the anterior maxilla: 3-year results of a case series on hard and soft tissue response and aesthetics. *J. Clin. Periodontol.* **2011**, *38*, 746–753. [CrossRef] [PubMed]
8. Galindo-Moreno, P.; Fernandez-Jimenez, A.; O'Valle, F.; Monje, A.; Silvestre, F.J.; Juodžbalys, G.; Sanchez-Fernandez, E.; Catena, A. Influence of the Crown-Implant Connection on the Preservation of Peri-Implant Bone: A Retrospective Multifactorial Analysis. *Int. J. Oral Maxillofac. Implant.* **2015**, *30*, 384–390. [CrossRef] [PubMed]
9. Lops, D.; Chiapasco, M.; Rossi, A.; Bressan, E.; Romeo, E. Incidence of inter-proximal papilla between a tooth and an adjacent immediate implant placed into a fresh extraction socket: 1-year prospective study. *Clin. Oral Implant. Res.* **2008**, *19*, 1135–1140. [CrossRef] [PubMed]
10. Lops, D.; Romeo, E.; Chiapasco, M.; Procopio, R.M.; Oteri, G. Behaviour of soft tissues healing around single bone-level-implants placed immediately after tooth extraction A 1 year prospective cohort study. *Clin. Oral Implant. Res.* **2012**, *24*, 1206–1213. [CrossRef] [PubMed]
11. Lops, D.; Parpaiola, A.; Paniz, G.; Sbricoli, L.; Magaz, V.; Venezze, A.; Bressan, E.; Stellini, E. Interproximal Papilla Stability Around CAD/CAM and Stock Abutments in Anterior Regions: A 2-Year Prospective Multicenter Cohort Study. *Int. J. Periodontics Restor. Dent.* **2017**, *37*, 657–665. [CrossRef] [PubMed]
12. Yotnuengnit, B.; Yotnuengnit, P.; Laohapand, P.; Athipanyakom, S. Emergence angles in natural anterior teeth: Influence on periodontal status. *Quintessence Int.* **2008**, *39*, e126–e133. [PubMed]
13. Mombelli, A.; Lang, N.P. Clinical parameters for the evaluation of dental implants. *Periodontol. 2000* **1994**, *4*, 81–86. [CrossRef] [PubMed]
14. Mombelli, A.; Lang, N.P. The diagnosis and treatment of peri-implantitis. *Periodontol. 2000* **1998**, *17*, 63–76. [CrossRef] [PubMed]
15. Inoue, M.; Nakano, T.; Shimomoto, T.; Kabata, D.; Shintani, A.; Yatani, H. Multivariate analysis of the influence of prosthodontic factors on peri-implant bleeding index and marginal bone level in a molar site: A cross-sectional study. *Clin. Implant Dent. Relat. Res.* **2020**, *22*, 713–722. [CrossRef] [PubMed]
16. Hentenaar, D.F.; De Waal, Y.C.; Van Winkelhoff, A.J.; Raghoebar, G.M.; Meijer, H.J. Influence of Cervical Crown Contour on Marginal Bone Loss Around Platform-Switched Bone-Level Implants: A 5-Year Cross-Sectional Study. *Int. J. Prosthodont.* **2020**, *33*, 373–379. [CrossRef] [PubMed]
17. Yi, Y.; Koo, K.; Schwarz, F.; Ben Amara, H.; Heo, S. Association of prosthetic features and peri-implantitis: A cross-sectional study. *J. Clin. Periodontol.* **2020**, *47*, 392–403. [CrossRef] [PubMed]
18. Degidi, M.; Daprile, G.; Piattelli, A. Marginal bone loss around implants with platform-switched Morse-cone connection: A radiographic cross-sectional study. *Clin. Oral Implant. Res.* **2016**, *28*, 1108–1112. [CrossRef] [PubMed]
19. Salina, S.; Gualini, F.; Rigotti, F.; Mazzarini, C.; Longhin, D.; Grigoletto, M.; Buti, J.; Sbricoli, L.; Esposito, M. Subcrestal placement of dental implants with an internal conical connection of 0.5 mm versus 1.5 mm: Three-year after loading results of a multicentre within-person randomised controlled trial. *Int. J. Oral Implant.* **2019**, *12*, 155–167.

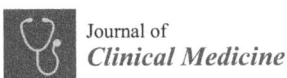

Article

Accuracy of a Computer-Aided Dynamic Navigation System in the Placement of Zygomatic Dental Implants: An In Vitro Study

Juan Ramón González Rueda [1], Irene García Ávila [1], Víctor Manuel de Paz Hermoso [2], Elena Riad Deglow [1], Álvaro Zubizarreta-Macho [1,3,*], Jesús Pato Mourelo [4], Javier Montero Martín [3] and Sofía Hernández Montero [1]

[1] Department of Implant Surgery, Faculty of Health Sciences, Alfonso X El Sabio University, 28691 Madrid, Spain; jgonzrue@myuax.com (J.R.G.R.); igarcavi@gmail.com (I.G.Á.); elenariaddeglow@gmail.com (E.R.D.); shernmon@uax.es (S.H.M.)
[2] Department of Maxillofacial Surgery, Quiron Health Hospital, 28002 Madrid, Spain; vdepaz@gmail.com
[3] Department of Surgery, Faculty of Medicine, University of Salamanca, 37008 Salamanca, Spain; javimont@usal.es
[4] Department of Surgery, Faculty of Dentistry, University of Navarra, 31009 Pamplona, Spain; jpatomourelo@hotmail.com
* Correspondence: amacho@uax.es

Abstract: The objective of this in vitro study was to evaluate and compare the accuracy of zygomatic dental implant (ZI) placement carried out using a dynamic navigation system. Materials and Methods: Forty (40) ZIs were randomly distributed into one of two study groups: (A) ZI placement via a computer-aided dynamic navigation system ($n = 20$) (navigation implant (NI)); and (B) ZI placement using a conventional free-hand technique ($n = 20$) (free-hand implant (FHI)). A cone-beam computed tomography (CBCT) scan of the existing situation was performed preoperatively to plan the surgical approach for the computer-aided study group. Four zygomatic dental implants were placed in anatomically based polyurethane models ($n = 10$) manufactured by stereolithography, and a postoperative CBCT scan was performed. Subsequently, the preoperative planning and postoperative CBCT scans were added to dental implant software to analyze the coronal entry point, apical end point, and angular deviations. Results were analyzed using the Student's *t*-test. Results: The results showed statistically significant differences in the apical end-point deviations between FHI and NI ($p = 0.0018$); however, no statistically significant differences were shown in the coronal entry point ($p = 0.2617$) or in the angular deviations ($p = 0.3132$). Furthermore, ZIs placed in the posterior region showed more deviations than the anterior region at the coronal entry point, apical end point, and angular level. Conclusions: The conventional free-hand technique enabled more accurate placement of ZIs than the computer-assisted surgical technique. In addition, placement of ZIs in the anterior region was more accurate than that in the posterior region.

Keywords: implantology; computer-aided surgery; image-guided surgery; zygomatic implants; navigation system

1. Introduction

Zygomatic implants (ZIs) have proven to be a suitable treatment option in the restoration of the extremely atrophic, totally edentulous maxillae usually caused by maxillary resection in patients with oncological pathologies, congenital deformities, or metabolic disorders—patients undergoing radiotherapy—or immunosuppressed patients [1]. ZIs are especially indicated for use in patients with compromised vascularization, which can affect the outcome of bone grafts used to regenerate maxillary defects; they are also indicated in cases of incompatibility of the donor area [2]. Specifically, ZIs provide a predictable treatment option that prevents long waiting times before prosthetic rehabilitation when compared with alternative techniques for conventional implant placement using grafting materials [3]. Additionally, a recent meta-analysis reported a failure rate of 2.89% (CI-95%

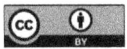

1.83–3.96%) associated with conventional-length dental implants ($n = 3549$), while the failed implantation of ZIs ($n = 1895$) had an estimated incidence rate of 0.69% (CI-95% 0.21–1.16%) over a follow-up period ranging from 3 to 163 months [4].

In 1988, Branemark first described using an intrasinusal placement approach for ZIs; however, this technique can lead to sinusitis, dental implant failure, oroantral fistula, periorbital and conjunctival hematoma or edema, paresthesia, difficulty speaking, pain, and edema [5]. Alternative placement approaches that depend on bone availability have subsequently emerged, such as the extrasinusal, extramaxillary, or slot techniques [6]; however, these are not devoid of intraoperative complications, which are primarily linked to operator experience. Therefore, preoperative planning techniques using cone-beam computed tomography (CBCT) scans [7] have been recommended to enable accurate computer-aided surgery with both static and dynamic navigation systems [8]. These increase the accuracy of dental implant placement, thereby reducing the risk of intraoperative complications and maintaining high survival rates of patients receiving dental implants [9]. Computer-aided surgery using static navigation systems has been widely used for the placement of conventional-length dental implants, showing a high success rate; furthermore, static navigation techniques have shown a mean horizontal deviation of 1.2 mm at the coronal entry point, 1.4 mm at the apical end point, and an angular deviation of 3.5° [10]. Computer-aided surgery using dynamic navigation systems has shown lower mean horizontal deviations at the coronal entry point (0.71 ± 0.40 mm), apical end point (1.00 ± 0.49 mm), and angular deviation ($2.26 \pm 1.62°$) [11]. Therefore, image-guided surgery approaches have been recommended to help increase the accuracy of ZI placement, preventing intraoperative and postoperative complications, as the length of ZIs is almost five times greater than a conventional-length dental implant; therefore, an entry-point or angular deviation of the dental implant bur may increase the apical-point deviation [12]. In addition, computer-aided surgery using dynamic navigation systems allows for free-hand implant navigation using high-precision motion tracking technology, preventing anatomical injuries [13]. Image-guided navigation systems also increase the accuracy of dental implant placement using artificial fiducial markers, which provide a virtual coordinate system linked to the surgical field or coordinate system of the patient [14]. However, computer-aided navigation systems are more expensive than surgical templates, and their accuracy depends on the learning curve and experience of the operator [15].

The objective of the present study was to evaluate the accuracy of placing ZIs using a dynamic navigation system. The null hypothesis (H0) stated that accuracy rates do not differ when comparing placement of ZIs using a dynamic navigation system versus a free-hand approach.

2. Materials and Methods

2.1. Study Design

This in vitro study was carried out between January and March 2021 at the Dental Center of Innovation and Advanced Specialties at Alfonso X El Sabio University in Madrid, Spain. The Ethical Committee of the Faculty of Health Sciences at Alfonso X El Sabio University approved the study in December 2020 (Process No. 25/2020). The patient gave their informed consent for the researchers to use their preoperative cone-beam computed tomography (CBCT) scan for the purposes of this study.

2.2. Experimental Procedure

Forty (40) ZIs (Galimplant, Sarria, Lugo, Spain) were planned and placed in teeth in positions 2.4 (4.3 mm × 30 mm, internal taper and conical wall), 2.2 (4.3 mm × 50 mm, internal taper and conical wall), 1.2 (4.3 mm × 52.5 mm, internal taper and conical wall), and 1.4 (4.3 mm × 35 mm, internal taper and conical wall). Researchers used an ANOVA to establish the sample size, achieving 80% power with a confidence level of 5%, with a variability between groups of 0.6 and an intragroup variability of 4, to identify differences in comparison with the null hypothesis H0: $\mu_1 = \mu_2 = \mu_3 = \mu_4$. Ten (10) anatomically based, standardized polyurethane models of a completely edentulous, atrophic, upper jaw maxilla were manufactured using a three-dimensional impression procedure (Sawbones Europe AB, Malmo, Sweden) based on a preoperative CBCT scan (WhiteFox, Satelec, Merignac, France). The scan was taken from a patient using the following exposure parameters: 8.0 mA, 105.0 kV peak, 7.20 s, with a 15 mm × 13 mm field of view (Figure 1). The anatomically based models were manufactured respecting the size and shape of the patient.

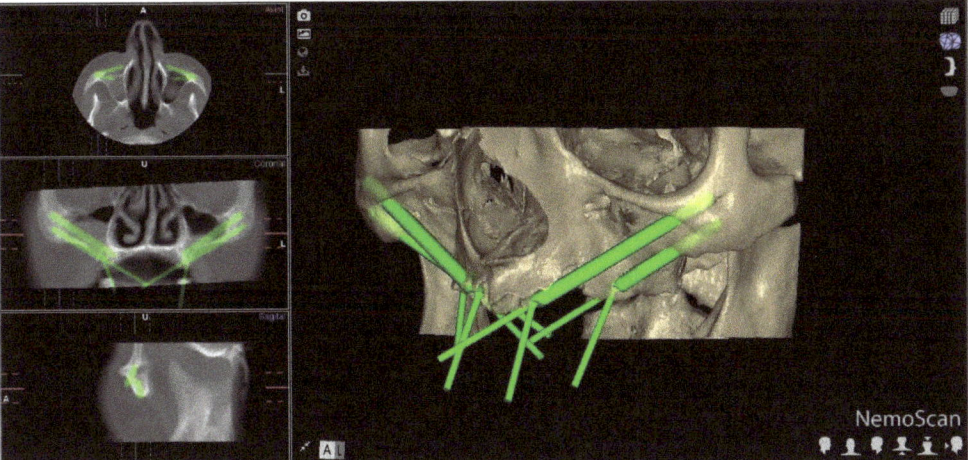

Figure 1. Preoperative planning of ZI placement based on the CBCT scan taken of the patient. Detail of the coronal, sagittal, and axial views, and three-dimensional reconstruction.

Afterwards, the models were fixed onto an artificial head to simulate the clinical conditions (Figure 2).

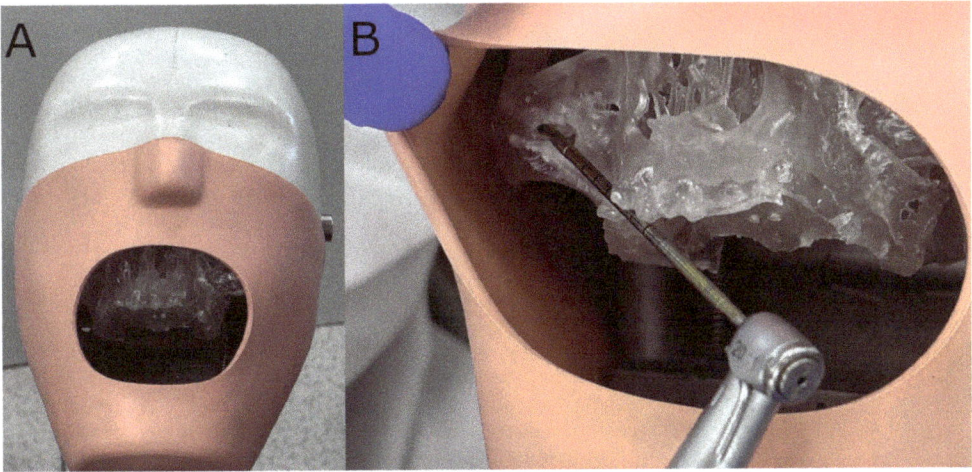

Figure 2. (**A**) Polyurethane model fixed onto an artificial head and (**B**) drilling procedure.

Researchers randomized the ZIs (Epidat 4.1, Galicia, Spain), which were assigned to one of two study groups: (A) ZI (Galimplant, Sarria, Lugo, Spain) placement using a computer-aided dynamic navigation system (Navident, ClaroNav, Toronto, ON, Canada)

(n = 20) (navigation implant (NI)); and (B) manual ZI (Galimplant, Sarria, Lugo, Spain) placement using a free-hand technique (n = 20) (freehand implant (FHI)). The order of placement of the ZIs (Galimplant, Sarria, Lugo, Spain) was randomized across the study groups (Epidat 4.1, Galicia, Spain), beginning with the NI study group and followed by the FHI control group.

A preoperative CBCT scan was taken of the NI anatomically based standardized polyurethane models (WhiteFox, Satelec, Merignac, France) prior to placing a jaw tag; the use of polyurethane was based on the American Society for Testing and Materials' (ASTM F-1839-08) approval of the use of polyurethane for testing instruments and dental implants ("Standard Specification for Rigid Polyurethane Foam for Use as a Standard Material for Test Orthopedic Devices for Instruments") [16]. This black-and-white tag was affixed to the dental surface of the anatomically based, standardized polyurethane models using a photopolymerized composite resin (Navistent, ClaroNav, Toronto, ON, Canada). The datasets obtained from the CBCT scan were uploaded to treatment-planning software (Navident, ClaroNav, Toronto, ON, Canada) on a laptop computer mounted onto a mobile unit to simulate placement of the ZIs in accordance with the prior surgical planning (Figure 3A). An additional black-and-white drill tag was affixed to the handpiece (W & H, Bürmoos, Austria). The researchers calibrated and identified both of the optical reference markers with an optical triangulation tracking system using stereoscopic motion-tracking cameras, orienting the drilling process in real time to ensure that the planned angle, pathway, and depth were achieved. A ZI system (Galimplant, Sarria, Lugo, Spain) was used to perform the drilling, with this procedure being monitored using the computer-aided dynamic navigation system installed onto the laptop computer (Figure 3B).

The conventional free-hand technique was used to place all ZIs (Galimplant, Sarria, Lugo, Spain) that had been randomly assigned to the FHI control group, with the operator having access to the preoperative planning and CBCT scan. All ZIs (Galimplant, Sarria, Lugo, Spain) were placed by a unique operator with prior surgical experience.

2.3. Measurement Procedure

Following placement of the ZIs, the researchers conducted postoperative CBCT scans (WhiteFox, Satelec, Merignac, France) using the aforementioned exposure parameters. The planning and postoperative CBCT scans (WhiteFox, Satelec, Merignac, France) of the different study groups were subsequently imported into 3D implant-planning software (NemoScan, Nemotec, Madrid, Spain). The scans were then overlaid in order to assess the apical deviation, measured at the coronal entry point (mm), apical end point (mm), and angular deviation (°), with the latter measured at the center of the cylinder. Any deviations that were noted in any of the implants were subsequently analyzed and compared between the axial, sagittal, and coronal views (Figure 4A–C) by an independent operator. In addition, deviations in the positions of the zygomatic dental implants were also recorded and analyzed.

2.4. Statistical Analysis

For each of the response variables, tables were produced with summaries of the following statistics according to group, position and group, and position: number of observations, mean, standard deviation, median, and the minimum and maximum values. These were represented graphically by box plots. Linear regression models with repeated measures were adjusted to analyze the differences according to group, according to position, and the interaction between both variables. Where statistically significant differences were detected, two-to-two comparisons were made between groups/positions. The p-values were adjusted using the Tukey method to correct the type I error. The statistical analysis was carried out using the software SAS v.9.4 (SAS Institute Inc., Cary, NC, USA). Statistical decisions were made using a significance level of 0.05.

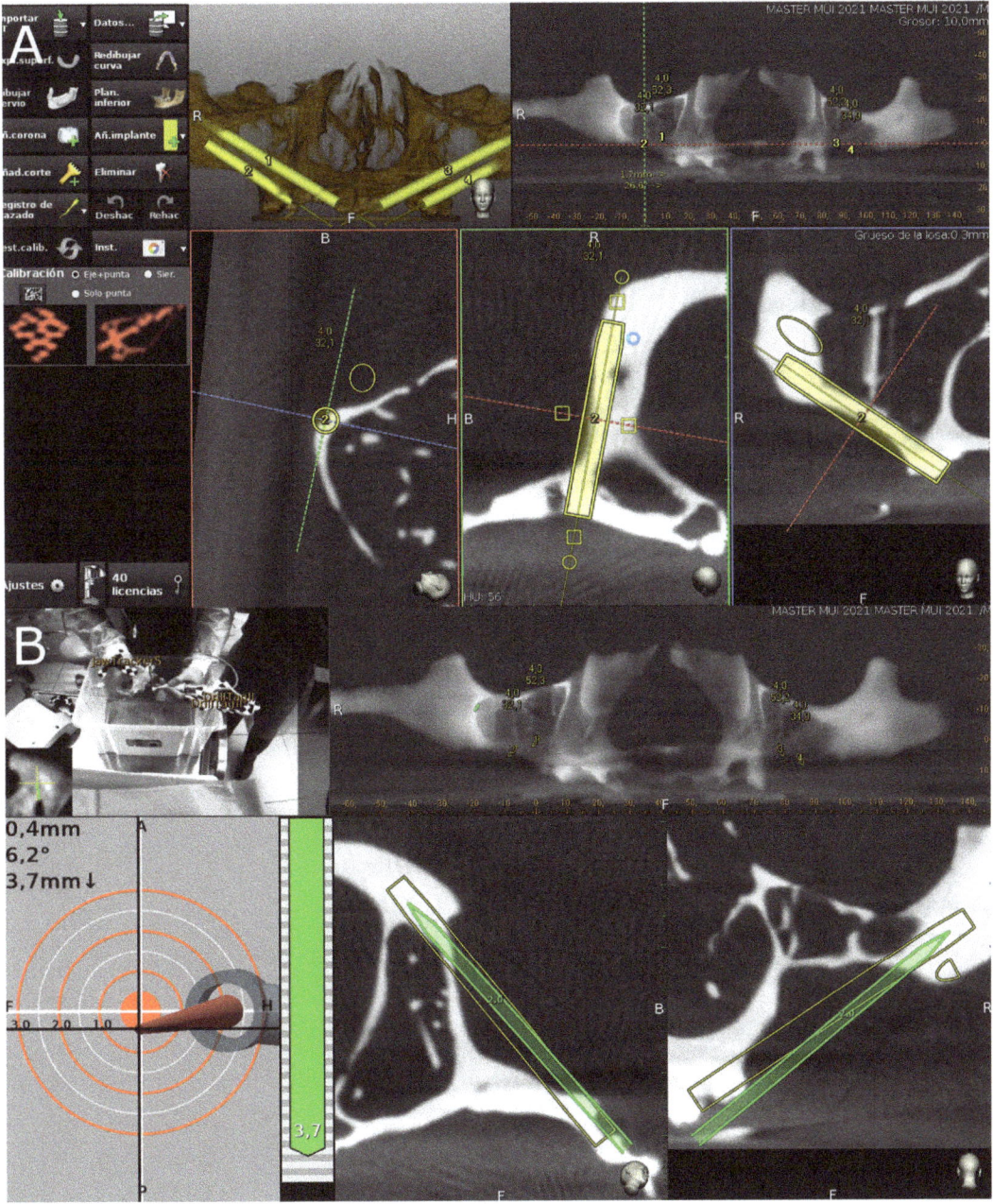

Figure 3. (**A**) Preoperative planning of placement of ZIs with the dynamic navigation appliance using treatment-planning software, and (**B**) tracking procedure during ZI placement.

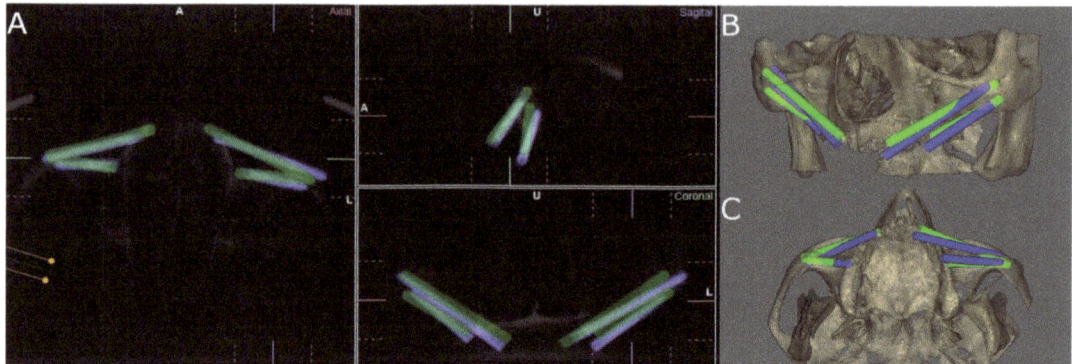

Figure 4. (**A**) CBCT images of the coronal, sagittal, and axial views; and (**B**) front and (**C**) bottom views of the three-dimensional reconstruction of the measurement procedure contrasted against the preoperative planning (green cylinders) and postoperative ZI placement (blue cylinders) of the ZIs placed on the experimental model.

3. Results

Table 1 shows the mean, median, and SD values with 95% confidence intervals for the coronal entry point (mm), apical end point (mm), and angular deviations (°) of the NI study group and the FHI control group.

Table 1. Descriptive values of deviations at the coronal entry point (mm), apical end point (mm), and angular (°) deviations of the computer-aided dynamic navigation technique (NI) and the free-hand approach.

		n	Mean	Median	SD	Lower 95% CL for Mean	Upper 95% CL for Mean	Minimum	Maximum
CORONAL	NI	19	5.43 [a]	5.70	2.13	4.41	6.46	1.60	10.50
	FHI	20	4.75 [a]	4.35	1.58	4.01	5.48	2.20	7.80
APICAL	NI	19	4.92 [a]	4.70	1.89	4.00	5.83	1.70	9.10
	FHI	20	3.20 [b]	3.30	1.45	2.52	3.88	0.60	5.40
ANGULAR	NI	19	7.36 [a]	6.20	4.12	5.37	9.34	0.90	16.10
	FHI	20	8.47 [b]	7.05	4.40	6.41	10.53	3.50	17.20

[a,b] Statistically significant differences ($p < 0.05$) found between groups. NI: navigation implants; and FHI: free-hand implants.

The paired Student's t-test did not find any statistically significant differences in the coronal entry-point deviations between the study groups ($p = 0.2617$), nor in the ZI positions ($p = 0.1649$). However, statistically significant deviations were observed between the computer-aided dynamic navigation technique (NI) and the free-hand approach at the ZI position 2.4 ($p = 0.0155$) (Figure 5).

The paired Student's t-test revealed statistically significant differences in the apical end-point deviations between the FHI control group and the NI study group ($p = 0.0018$). On the other hand, no statistically significant differences were observed between the zygomatic dental implant positions ($p = 0.1856$), except at the ZI position 2.4 ($p = 0.0005$) (Figure 6).

The paired Student's t-test found no statistically significant differences between the angular deviations of the study groups ($p = 0.3132$); on the other hand, statistically significant differences were shown for the zygomatic dental implant positions ($p = 0.0008$), especially at the ZI position 1.4 ($p = 0.0040$) (Figure 7).

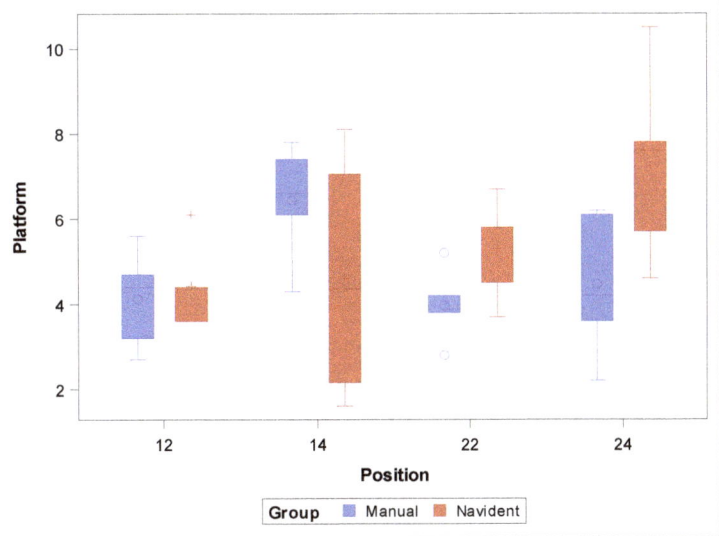

Figure 5. Box plot of deviations at the coronal entry point observed in the study groups and ZI positions. Median values are represented by the horizontal lines within each box. The symbols represent extreme values.

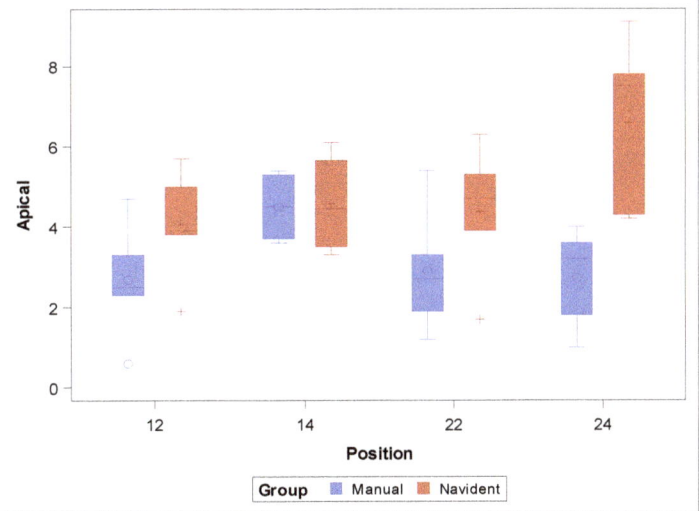

Figure 6. Box plot of apical end-point deviations recorded in the study groups and ZI positions. Median values are represented by the horizontal lines within each box. The symbols represent extreme values.

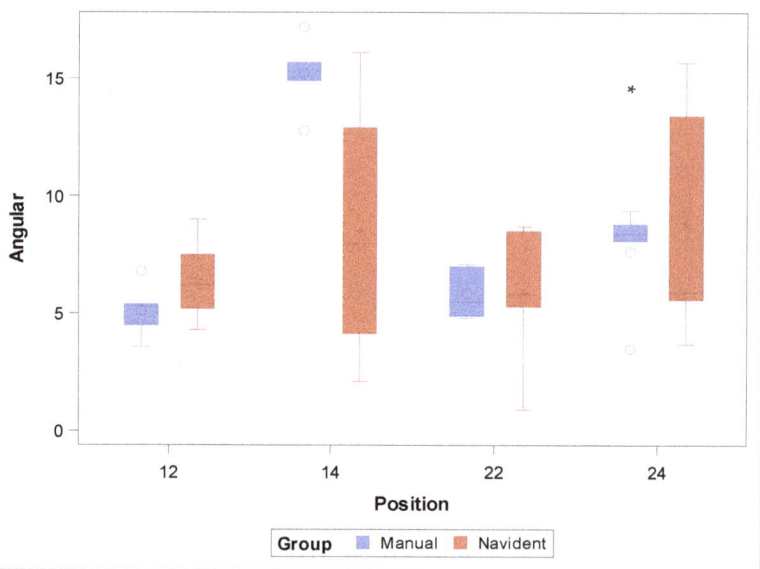

Figure 7. Box plot of angular deviations found in the study groups and ZI positions. Median values are represented by the horizontal lines within each box. The symbols represent extreme values.

In summary, the FHI approach showed lower deviation values at the coronal entry point and the apical end point. This may be because the ZIs assigned to the FHI control group were the last to be placed, enabling the operator to learn and to memorize the correct position of the ZI. Furthermore, ZIs placed in posterior regions showed higher levels of deviation at the coronal entry point, apical end point, and angular level.

One ZI was withdrawn from the NI study group because the osteotomy site preparations did not provide sufficient stability for the ZI.

4. Discussion

The results of the present study reject the null hypothesis (H0), which states that there is no difference in accuracy when comparing placement of ZIs using a dynamic navigation system versus a free-hand approach.

The primary findings of the present study indicate that the free-hand conventional technique for ZI placement was more accurate than the computer-aided dynamic navigation technique at the coronal and apical levels; however, the computer-aided dynamic navigation technique showed more accuracy than the free-hand conventional technique at the angular level.

Hung et al. [17], Xiaojun et al. [18], Chen et al. [19], Hung et al. [20], Zhu et al. [8], and Jorba-García et al. [21] found computer-aided dynamic navigation to have greater accuracy than the free-hand conventional approach for the placement of conventional-length dental implants. Nevertheless, Brief et al. found that, although computer-aided navigation techniques are significantly more accurate than free-hand conventional techniques, the level of accuracy provided by the free-hand conventional technique is sufficient for most clinical situations [22]. However, Aydemir et al. reported that the conventional free-hand technique provides greater accuracy at the coronal entry-point and apical end-point levels than the computer-assisted dynamic navigation technique in the placement of ZIs, although the computer-aided dynamic navigation technique resulted in lower angular deviation than the free-hand conventional technique [23]. Moreover, Jung et al. found similar safety levels, outcomes, morbidity, and efficiency between computer-aided navigation techniques and free-hand conventional techniques for placement of conventional-length dental implants [24]. These results corroborate those of the present study, and the learning curve required for the use of computer-aided dynamic navigation systems may explain the discrepancies observed between the dynamic navigation system and the free-hand conventional technique [11]. Additionally, Mediavilla Guzmán et al. warned of low methodological quality in the studies related to ZIs, which makes it difficult to compare the results of the different studies [13]. Gunkel et al. also found that studies conducted under laboratory or in vitro conditions showed higher accuracy rates than clinical studies [25]. Likewise, Kim et al. [26] and Tahmaseb et al. [27] reported variability in the accuracy of computer-aided surgery using static navigation systems, depending on the study design.

Otherwise, Jorba-García et al. showed a mean angular deviation of 2.1° and a mean horizontal deviation of 0.46 mm at the coronal entry point for computer-aided surgery using dynamic navigation systems [28]. Xiaojun et al. showed a mean horizontal deviation of 1.36 ± 0.59 mm at the coronal entry point of conventional-length dental implants [18]; Chen et al., 1.12 ± 0.29 mm [14]; Hung et al., 1.07 ± 0.15 mm [20]; Hung et al., 1.35 ± 0.75 mm [17]; Block et al., 0.4 mm [29]; Kaewsiri et al., 1.05 ± 0.44 mm [30]; and Zhou et al., 1.56 ± 0.54 mm [8]. However, the present study showed a higher mean horizontal deviation at the coronal entry point (5.43 ± 2.13 mm), possibly due to the learning curve and operator experience. Kaewsiri et al. reported a mean horizontal deviation of 1.29 ± 0.50 mm at the apical end point, directly correlated with the length of the dental implant (8, 10, and 12 mm) [30]. Consequently, the horizontal deviation at the apical end point would be higher in ZIs than in conventional-length dental implants. In addition, Chrcanovic et al. reported an anteroposterior angular deviation of $8.06 \pm 6.40°$ and craniocaudal of $11.20 \pm 9.75°$, which led to the invasion of the infratemporal fossa and the orbit by the ZIs [31]. Moreover, Vrielinck et al. found a mean angular deviation of 5.1° (ranging from 0.8 to 9.0° [32]; Xiaojun et al., $4.1 \pm 0.9°$ [18]; Zhou et al., $2.52 \pm 0.84°$ [8]; Hung et al., $1.37 \pm 0.21°$ [17]; Hung et al., $2.05 \pm 1.02°$ [20]; and Chen et al., $0.19 \pm 0.92°$ [14]. These results are slightly lower than those obtained in the present study ($7.36 \pm 4.12°$). These deviation values may lead to clinical and/or prosthetic complications in 36.4% of ZI placements, primarily due to a lack of primary stability [33]. In the present study, one ZI randomly placed using the dynamic navigation system was also removed due to insufficient stability at the prepared osteotomy site. In addition, Lan et al. described all complications related to the ZI placement procedure, reporting a malposition rate of 12% (95% confidence interval [CI]: 4 to 23%), surgical guiding failure rate of 11% (95% CI: 3 to 21%), and local infection/injury rate of 10% (95% CI: 3 to 18%) [34]. Additionally, Gutiérrez et al. reported that the prosthetic rehabilitations of ZIs have shown a low incidence of prosthetic complications (4.9% (95% CI: 2.7–7.3%)), regardless of the prosthetic treatment. The present study also found that the ZI placed in position 2.4 showed statistically significant deviations at the coronal entry point, and the ZI placed in position 1.4 showed statistically significant deviations in angular deviation. In summary, the ZIs placed in the anterior region showed lower deviations than the ZIs placed in the posterior region, likely due to better accessibility and visibility of the operative field.

The findings of the present study can be useful to clinicians in selecting the more accurate technique for ZI placement in patients with atrophied maxilla who must undergo full-arch rehabilitation by means of ZIs. The authors recommend improving the methodological quality of studies and increasing the body of evidence by way of additional randomized studies implementing new computer-assisted navigation techniques.

5. Conclusions

Within the limitations of the present study, the results indicated that the free-hand conventional technique provided greater accuracy in the placement of ZIs than the computer-assisted surgical technique. In addition, placement of ZIs in the anterior region was more accurate than that in the posterior region.

Author Contributions: Conceptualization, J.R.G.R., I.G.Á. and Á.Z.-M.; design, V.M.d.P.H.; data acquisition, E.R.D.; formal analysis, J.P.M.; statistical analyses, Á.Z.-M. and S.H.M.; review and editing, J.M.M. All authors have read and agreed to the published version of the manuscript.

Funding: This research received no external funding.

Institutional Review Board Statement: Not applicable.

Informed Consent Statement: Not applicable.

Data Availability Statement: Data are available on request, pursuant to any applicable restrictions (e.g., ethical or privacy considerations).

Conflicts of Interest: The authors declare no conflict of interest.

References

1. Bidra, A.S.; Jacob, R.F.; Taylor, T.D. Classification of maxillectomy defects: A systematic review and criteria necessary for a universal description. *J. Prosthet. Dent.* **2012**, *107*, 261–270. [CrossRef]
2. Rosenstein, J.; Dym, H. Zygomatic Implants: A Solution for the Atrophic Maxilla. *Dent. Clin. N. Am.* **2020**, *64*, 401–409. [CrossRef] [PubMed]
3. Davó, R.; Felice, P.; Pistilli, R.; Barausse, C.; Marti-Pages, C.; Ferrer-Fuertes, A.; Ippolito, D.R.; Esposito, M. Immediately loaded zygomatic implants vs. conventional dental implants in augmented atrophic maxillae: 1-year post-loading results from a multicentre randomised controlled trial. *Eur. J. Oral Implantol.* **2018**, *11*, 145–161. [PubMed]
4. Gutiérrez Muñoz, D.; Obrador Aldover, C.; Zubizarreta-Macho, Á.; González Menéndez, H.; Lorrio Castro, J.; Peñarrocha-Oltra, D.; Montiel-Company, J.M.; Hernández Montero, S. Survival Rate and Prosthetic and Sinus Complications of Zygomatic Dental Implants for the Rehabilitation of the Atrophic Edentulous Maxilla: A Systematic Review and Meta-Analysis. *Biology* **2021**, *10*, 601. [CrossRef] [PubMed]
5. Brånemark, P.I.; Gröndahl, K.; Ohrnell, L.O.; Nilsson, P.; Petruson, B.; Svensson, B.; Engstrand, P.; Nannmark, U. Zygoma fixture in the management of advanced atrophy of the maxilla: Technique and long-term results. *Scand. J. Plast. Reconstr. Surg. Hand Surg.* **2004**, *38*, 70–85. [CrossRef] [PubMed]
6. Maló, P.; Nobre Mde, A.; Lopes, I. A new approach to rehabilitate the severely atrophic maxilla using extramaxillary anchored implants in immediate function: A pilot study. *J. Prosthet. Dent.* **2008**, *100*, 354–366. [CrossRef]
7. Omami, G.; Al Yafi, F. Should Cone Beam Computed Tomography Be Routinely Obtained in Implant Planning? *Dent. Clin. N. Am.* **2019**, *63*, 363–379. [CrossRef]
8. Zhou, W.; Fan, S.; Wang, F.; Huang, W.; Jamjoom, F.Z.; Wu, Y. A novel extraoral registration method for a dynamic navigation system guiding zygomatic implant placement in patients with maxillectomy defects. *Int. J. Oral Maxillofac. Surg.* **2021**, *50*, 116–120. [CrossRef]
9. Chana, H.; Smith, G.; Bansal, H.; Zahra, D. A Retrospective Cohort Study of the Survival Rate of 88 Zygomatic Implants Placed Over an 18-year Period. *Int. J. Oral Maxillofac. Implants* **2019**, *34*, 461–470. [CrossRef]
10. Tahmaseb, A.; Wu, V.; Wismeijer, D.; Coucke, W.; Evans, C. The accuracy of static computer-aided implant surgery: A systematic review and meta-analysis. *Clin. Oral Implants Res.* **2018**, *16*, 416–435. [CrossRef]
11. Stefanelli, L.V.; DeGroot, B.S.; Lipton, D.I.; Mandelaris, G.A. Accuracy of a Dynamic Dental Navigation System in a Private Practice. *Int. J. Oral Maxillofac. Implants* **2019**, *34*, 205–213. [CrossRef] [PubMed]
12. Wu, Y.; Wang, F.; Huang, W.; Fan, S. Real-Time Navigation in Zygomatic Implant Placement: Workflow. *Oral Maxillofac. Surg. Clin. N. Am.* **2019**, *31*, 357–367. [CrossRef] [PubMed]
13. Mediavilla Guzmán, A.; Riad Deglow, E.; Zubizarreta-Macho, Á.; Agustín-Panadero, R.; Hernández Montero, S. Accuracy of Computer-Aided Dynamic Navigation Compared to Computer-Aided Static Navigation for Dental Implant Placement: An In Vitro Study. *J. Clin. Med.* **2019**, *8*, 2123. [CrossRef] [PubMed]
14. Chen, C.K.; Yuh, D.Y.; Huang, R.Y.; Fu, E.; Tsai, C.F.; Chiang, C.Y. Accuracy of Implant Placement with a Navigation System, a Laboratory Guide, and Freehand Drilling. *Int. J. Oral Maxillofac. Implants* **2018**, *33*, 1213–1218. [CrossRef]
15. Gargallo-Albiol, J.; Barootchi, S.; Salomó-Coll, O.; Wang, H.L. Advantages and disadvantages of implant navigation surgery. A systematic review. *Ann. Anat.* **2019**, *225*, 1–10. [CrossRef]
16. Comuzzi, L.; Tumedei, M.; Pontes, A.E.; Piattelli, A.; Iezzi, G. Primary Stability of Dental Implants in Low-Density (10 and 20 pcf) Polyurethane Foam Blocks: Conical vs. Cylindrical Implants. *Int. J. Environ. Res. Public Health* **2020**, *17*, 2617. [CrossRef]
17. Hung, K.F.; Wang, F.; Wang, H.W.; Zhou, W.J.; Huang, W.; Wu, Y.Q. Accuracy of a real-time surgical navigation system for the placement of quad zygomatic implants in the severe atrophic maxilla: A pilot clinical study. *Clin. Implant Dent. Relat. Res.* **2017**, *19*, 458–465. [CrossRef]
18. Xiaojun, C.; Ming, Y.; Yanping, L.; Yiqun, W.; Chengtao, W. Image guided oral implantology and its application in the placement of zygoma implants. *Comput. Methods Programs Biomed.* **2009**, *93*, 162–173. [CrossRef]
19. Chen, X.; Wu, Y.; Wang, C. Application of a surgical navigation system in the rehabilitation of maxillary defects using zygoma implants: Report of one case. *Int. J. Oral Maxillofac. Implants* **2011**, *26*, e29–e34.

20. Hung, K.; Huang, W.; Wang, F.; Wu, Y. Real-Time Surgical Navigation System for the Placement of Zygomatic Implants with Severe Bone Deficiency. *Int. J. Oral Maxillofac. Implants* **2016**, *31*, 1444–1449. [CrossRef]
21. Jorba-García, A.; Figueiredo, R.; González-Barnadas, A.; Camps-Font, O.; Valmaseda-Castellón, E. Accuracy and the role of experience in dynamic computer guided dental implant surgery: An in-vitro study. *Med. Oral Patol. Oral Cir. Bucal.* **2019**, *24*, e76–e83. [CrossRef] [PubMed]
22. Brief, J.; Edinger, D.; Hassfeld, S.; Eggers, G. Accuracy of image-guided implantology. *Clin. Oral Implants Res.* **2005**, *16*, 495–501. [CrossRef] [PubMed]
23. Aydemir, C.A.; Arısan, V. Accuracy of dental implant placement via dynamic navigation or the freehand method: A split-mouth randomized controlled clinical trial. *Clin. Oral Implants Res.* **2020**, *31*, 255–263. [CrossRef] [PubMed]
24. Jung, R.E.; Schneider, D.; Ganeles, J.; Wismeijer, D.; Zwahlen, M.; Hämmerle, C.H.; Tahmaseb, A. Computer technology applications in surgical implant dentistry: A systematic review. *Int. J. Oral Maxillofac. Implants* **2009**, *24*, 92–109.
25. Gunkel, A.R.; Freysinger, W.; Thumfart, W.F. Experience with various 3-dimensional navigation systems in head and neck surgery. *Arch. Otolaryngol. Head Neck Surg.* **2000**, *126*, 390–395. [CrossRef] [PubMed]
26. Kim, S.G.; Lee, W.J.; Lee, S.S.; Heo, M.S.; Huh, K.H.; Choi, S.C.; Kim, T.I.; Yi, W.J. An advanced navigational surgery system for dental implants completed in a single visit: An in vitro study. *J. Craniomaxillofac. Surg.* **2015**, *43*, 117–125. [CrossRef] [PubMed]
27. Tahmaseb, A.; Wismeijer, D.; Coucke, W.; Derksen, W. Computer technology applications in surgical implant dentistry: A systematic review. *Int. J. Oral Maxillofac. Implants* **2014**, *29*, 25–42. [CrossRef]
28. Jorba-García, A.; González-Barnadas, A.; Camps-Font, O.; Figueiredo, R.; Valmaseda-Castellón, E. Accuracy assessment of dynamic computer-aided implant placement: A systematic review and meta-analysis. *Clin Oral Investig.* **2021**, *25*, 2479–2494. [CrossRef]
29. Block, M.S.; Emery, R.W.; Lank, K.; Ryan, J. Implant Placement Accuracy Using Dynamic Navigation. *Int. J. Oral Maxillofac. Implants* **2017**, *32*, 92–99. [CrossRef]
30. Kaewsiri, D.; Panmekiate, S.; Subbalekha, K.; Mattheos, N.; Pimkhaokham, A. The accuracy of static vs. dynamic computer-assisted implant surgery in single tooth space: A randomized controlled trial. *Clin. Oral Implants Res.* **2019**, *30*, 505–514. [CrossRef]
31. Chrcanovic, B.R.; Oliveira, D.R.; Custódio, A.L. Accuracy evaluation of computed tomography-derived stereolithographic surgical guides in zygomatic implant placement in human cadavers. *J. Oral Implantol.* **2010**, *36*, 345–355. [CrossRef] [PubMed]
32. Vrielinck, L.; Politis, C.; Schepers, S.; Pauwels, M.; Naert, I. Image-based planning and clinical validation of zygoma and pterygoid implant placement in patients with severe bone atrophy using customized drill guides. Preliminary results from a prospective clinical follow-up study. *Int. J. Oral Maxillofac. Surg.* **2003**, *32*, 7–14. [CrossRef] [PubMed]
33. Ramezanzade, S.; Yates, J.; Tuminelli, F.J.; Keyhan, S.O.; Yousefi, P.; Lopez-Lopez, J. Zygomatic implants placed in atrophic maxilla: An overview of current systematic reviews and meta-analysis. *Maxillofac. Plast. Reconstr. Surg.* **2021**, *43*, 1. [CrossRef] [PubMed]
34. Lan, K.; Wang, F.; Huang, W.; Davó, R.; Wu, Y. Quad Zygomatic Implants: A Systematic Review and Meta-analysis on Survival and Complications. *Int. J. Oral Maxillofac. Implants* **2021**, *36*, 21–29. [CrossRef] [PubMed]

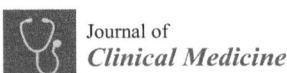

Article

A Retrospective Digital Analysis of Contour Changing after Tooth Extraction with or without Using Less Traumatic Surgical Procedures

Giovanni Battista Menchini-Fabris [1,2,3,*], Paolo Toti [1,4], Roberto Crespi [1,2], Giovanni Crespi [1], Saverio Cosola [1] and Ugo Covani [1,4]

1 Department of Stomatology, Tuscan Stomatologic Institute, Foundation for Dental Clinic, Research and Continuing Education, 55041 Camaiore, Italy; capello.totipaolo@gmail.com (P.T.); robcresp@libero.it (R.C.); gio.crespi@hotmail.it (G.C.); s.cosola@hotmail.it (S.C.); covani@covani.it (U.C.)
2 Study Center for Multidisciplinary Regenerative Research, Guglielmo Marconi University, 00100 Rome, Italy
3 San Rossore Dental Unit, Viale delle Cascine 152, San Rossore, 56122 Pisa, Italy
4 Department of Dentistry, Unicamillus—Saint Camillus International University of Health and Medical Sciences, 00100 Rome, Italy
* Correspondence: editorial.activities@istitutostomatologicotoscano.it; Tel.: +39-339-715-7007 or +39-050-578815

Citation: Menchini-Fabris, G.B.; Toti, P.; Crespi, R.; Crespi, G.; Cosola, S.; Covani, U. A Retrospective Digital Analysis of Contour Changing after Tooth Extraction with or without Using Less Traumatic Surgical Procedures. *J. Clin. Med.* 2022, 11, 922. https://doi.org/10.3390/jcm11040922

Academic Editors: Giulia Brunello and Adolfo Di Fiore

Received: 7 January 2022
Accepted: 8 February 2022
Published: 10 February 2022

Publisher's Note: MDPI stays neutral with regard to jurisdictional claims in published maps and institutional affiliations.

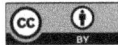

Copyright: © 2022 by the authors. Licensee MDPI, Basel, Switzerland. This article is an open access article distributed under the terms and conditions of the Creative Commons Attribution (CC BY) license (https://creativecommons.org/licenses/by/4.0/).

Abstract: Background: The present retrospective analysis aimed to compare two different single tooth extraction surgical approaches in both premolar and molar areas: less traumatic magneto-electrical versus conventional tooth extraction in minimizing the edentulous ridge volume loss. Methods: In the present retrospective control trial, 48 patients who underwent one-tooth extraction, were allocated either to control (28 sites treated with conventional tooth extraction procedures) or test group (20 subjects treated with less traumatic tooth extraction procedures by tooth sectioning and magnetoelectric roots subluxation). Intraoperatively (during tooth extraction surgery just after the subsequent filling of the alveolar socket with the sterile fast re-absorbable gelatin sponge), and then four months later, contours of the sockets were acquired through a laser intra-oral scanner. The digitally superimposed models were converted to dicom (Digital Imaging and Communications in Medicine) format first, then volumetric and area evaluations were performed with a DentaScan tool package. Non-parametric tests were applied with a level of significance set at $p < 0.01$. Results: significant reductions of anatomical features were observed four months later in all the groups (p-values < 0.001) with volume losses leading to a final alveolar ridge volume of 0.87 ± 0.34 cm^3 for atraumatic extractions and 0.66 ± 0.19 cm^3 for conventional extractions. No significant differences were registered for outcomes related to the basal surface variables. When just molar tooth were considered, the outcomes relating to volume loss between baseline and four months (ΔV) and its percentage ($\Delta V\%$) showed a better behavior in the less traumatic procedure ($\Delta V = -0.30 \pm 0.10$ cm^3 and $\Delta V\% = -22.3 \pm 8.4\%$) compared to the conventional extractions ($\Delta V = -0.59 \pm 0.10$ cm^3 and $\Delta V\% = -44.3 \pm 5.8\%$) with p-values < 0.0001. Conclusions: at four months, the less traumatic tooth extraction procedures by tooth sectioning and magnetoelectric root subluxation seemed to be able to better preserve the volume of the alveolar crest (reduction close to 22% with less traumatic extraction in molar sites) when compared to subjects treated with the conventional tooth extraction techniques.

Keywords: alveolar remodeling; tooth extraction; intraoral digital scanning; imaging superimposition; less traumatic surgery; socket healing

1. Introduction

It was well known that to place a dental implant reaching an acceptable aesthetics of prosthetic restoration, it was fundamental to manage the alveolar bone remodeling after tooth extraction by counteracting the reduction of width and height of the alveolar ridge [1–3].

The remodeling of hard and soft tissues could be affected by many different factors, such as the anatomical features of the extraction sites, all the other treatments following the extraction surgery, and obviously, any surgical procedure or tooth extraction technique as well [4–7].

To minimize any negative impact of the tooth removal procedure to the alveolar socket healing, several instruments had been introduced and used during the so-called Less Traumatic Extraction Techniques" (LTETs) such as forceps, periotomes, and luxators, along with piezosurgical, magnetoelectrical, and root extraction system devices [8].

Conventional extraction surgery consisted in using the elevators and forceps, which could easily damage the coronal aspect of the buccal and palatal/lingual cortical bone of the alveolar crest; this occurred if shattered root fragments had to be removed with the reflection of a mucoperiosteal flap, with the removal of bone to retrieve roots, and by utilizing tooth movement in a horizontal direction or by rotating it till to root(s) luxation [9,10].

In this respect, elevators could pull out the tooth from a socket by using adjacent bone margins acting as fulcra [11]. This high extractive force used could cause severe soft and hard tissue trauma [12].

When more aggressive surgeries had to be used, i.e., for multi-rooted teeth with ankilotic or divergent roots, different minimally invasive procedures that applied a mechanical strength rather than using the force of the surgeon had been described [13].

In this view, any damage caused to the facial bone wall of the alveolar socket at the time of extraction could influence the loss in width and height of the alveolar ridge during the healing period. They were, precisely, the piezosurgical devices and vibrating syndesmotomes that gently acted to sever the cervical fibers of the periodontal ligament surrounding the tooth between the root and socket. So, all this ensured that the coronal tissues of the extraction socket did not undergo any traumatic ripping [14,15].

The alveolar shrinkage after tooth extraction was so well known that clinicians devised several methods for maintaining or augmenting the ridge volume waiting for delayed implant placement [16,17]. Different grafting materials and techniques were recommended to preserve the alveolar ridge during the healing phase [18–20]. However, a clinician who was very careful when handling the tissues rounding a tooth to be extracted played an important part in the alveolar ridge preservation.

The concept behind root extraction systems was that a single root could be pulled out in its axial direction with precision given by the several proposed corkscrew devices without any direct trauma to the socket walls [21]. This strategy was of particular relevance in single-rooted teeth (anterior maxilla and mandible). On the contrary, since no extractions of teeth in posterior sites could adversely affect aesthetic outcomes, it was reported that the buccal contour of the alveolar ridge underwent 50% volume loss within one year after surgery [1].

A less traumatic tooth extraction could be performed by the clinician even without the aid of any device or new technology. As said, electromagnetic dental mallet helped reduce tissues damage in implant prosthetic rehabilitation as suggested by Crespi and co-workers [22]. A midcourse between very less traumatic devices and surgeon manual intervention could be the use of mechanical periotomes that advanced apically with minimal hand pressure in a quick and precise way and without any effort of the clinicians in extracting teeth [23].

Three-dimensional digital systems employed in the rehabilitation workflow, such as digital models as an alternative to plaster casts, represented an important technological advancement allowing identification of better surgical procedures and translating the adoption of more effective therapies [24,25]. Stereolithographic (.stl) model allowed the clinicians to calculate the changes guaranteeing high levels of accuracy when different .stl point clouds had to be superimposed [16,26]. This could be carried out semi-automatically with the help of a clinician (via triangulation of the occlusal planes) [27].

The primary aim of the present retrospective analysis was to test the effectiveness of two types of posterior single tooth extraction (less traumatic magneto-electrical versus conventional tooth extraction) in maintaining contour stability of the socket area; sockets were observed using an intraoral laser scanner that provided three-dimensional digital models of the patients' dental arches acquired intraoperatively (just after tooth extraction) and then four months after the first surgery. A secondary aim was to test if a loss in the contour of the edentulous area depended on the extracted tooth site (bicuspids versus molars).

2. Materials and Methods

2.1. Study Design/Sample

Case sheets of patients treated for tooth extraction from 2016 to 2019 were gathered to access patients' personal information. Collected schedules were reviewed to extract useful information and relevant data.

Patients inclusion criteria:

- 18 years old or older;
- signed and informed consent form for data processing;
- single intercalate tooth extraction in the back area (bicuspid and molar teeth);
- presence of an uncorrupted dataset of two three-dimensional scans (file.stl) in the collected records, representing intraoperative views on just treated sites (acquired during tooth extraction surgery just after the filling of the alveolar socket with a sterile fast re-absorbable gelatin sponge) and on healed postsurgical areas (around 4 months later).

Patients exclusion criteria:

- history of systemic diseases contraindicating oral surgical intervention;
- any report for bisphosphonate therapy;
- history of bone resection or radiation therapy (as part of an oncological treatment);
- lost or corrupted .stl file of the virtual models.

Patients were intra- and postoperatively scanned with a 25 µm precision 3-dimensional optical scanner (TRIOS 3, 3Shape A/S, Holmens Kanal, Copenhagen, Denmark).

A matrix elaborator (MatLab 7.11, The MathWorks, Natick, MA, USA) read information from .stl files and processed data of two full-arch digital models. For each patient, digital stereolithographic files were voxelized; the process of voxelization consisted of converting the .stl vertices into the same number of voxels to create 16-bit three-dimensional clouds; their primary characteristic was that they could be easily read on the dentascan (list in Appendix A). The two voxelized clouds were superimposed each other by using a best-fit algorithm as described and listed by Menchini-Fabris and co-workers to occupy the same space at the same time; the position of each digital model was triangulated from its occlusal surface given by the remaining teeth to be exact [27]; then the matrices were fused each other by another subroutine (list in Appendix B).

Results were saved as dicom images by applying the following setting: Field Of View = 10.24 cm, isometric voxel = 100 µm.

Dicom images with fused full-arch digital models underwent volume and surface measurements in a dedicated dentascan software (SimPlant 12.02, Materialise Dental Italia, Roma, Italy) as per Crespi and colleague [28].

The boundaries of the standardized Volume Of Interest (VOI) were defined as the following. VOI domain was a parallelepiped with six faces: mesial and distal border walls were perpendicular to both a cross-sectional line passing in the middle of the alveolar ridge and the occlusal plane, and they were tangential to the remaining teeth surfaces towards the edentulous area (distal crown surface of the anterior tooth and mesial crown surface of the posterior tooth, respectively); buccal/palatal border walls were perpendicular to both the mesial and the distal walls, as well as to the occlusal plane; basal/coronal walls were perpendicular to all the others being, respectively, the base and the cover of the VOI box. Coronal boundary stretched from the most coronal point of preoperative papillae to the level of 10 mm toward the apical direction, which corresponded to the basal plane (or surface). A graphical representation of the VOI was shown in Figure 1.

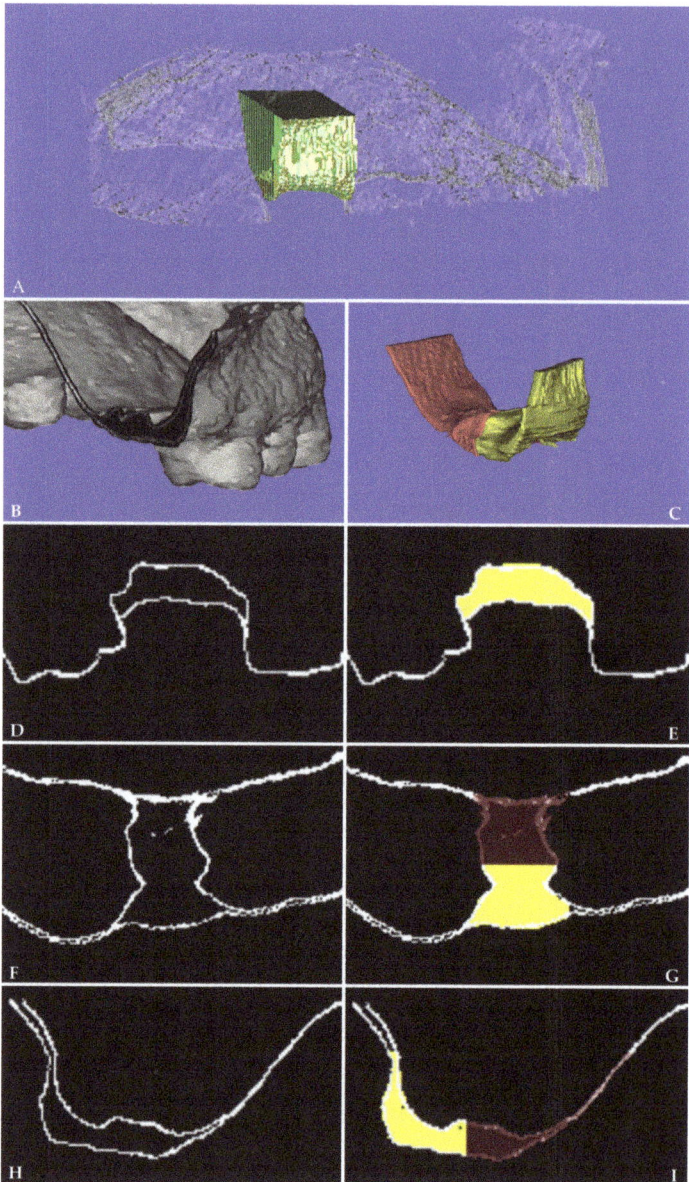

Figure 1. Buccal and palatal volume measurements (**A**) Three-dimensional voxelized .stl cloud with measured alveolar ridge volume at T0 (in green) and basal surface (in dark green) within the Volume Of Interest, (**B**) isometric rendering of two fused voxelized .stl clouds (intraoperative versus 4-month survey) with (**C**) view of the change of alveolar ridge volume, buccal (in yellow) and palatal (in red). (**D**,**E**) sagittal, (**F**,**G**) axial, and (**H**,**I**) cross-sectional views of the clouds obtained by an intraoral optical scanner.

Then, a single-blind examiner and collector (TP) performed all volume and area measurements using the "prepare for planning" toolbox of the dentascan.

2.2. Surgery Procedures

One hour before surgery, patients were treated with "one-shot" antibiotic administration as a pre-medication (2 g amoxicillin or 0.6 g. of clindamycin for subjects allergic to penicillins and cephalosporins). After a mouth rinse with 0.2% chlorhexidine for 1 min, patients were treated under local anesthesia using lidocaine with epinephrine (1:50,000).

Less traumatic tooth extraction

The tooth was extracted with the maximum preservation of the hard and soft tissue with the least traumatic procedure as possible. The way was to pull out each tooth just like a single-rooted one. When multi-rooted, the tooth required a surgical crown sectioning with one root per crown segment, on the other hand in the cases of fused or convergent roots, sectioning was not required. Neither flaps were raised nor releasing incisions performed. When necessary periotomes were used to sever the cervical gingival attachment fibers. Extraction was performed using an electromagnetic device (Magnetic Mallet, www.osseotouch.com (accessed on 6 January 2022), Turbigo, Milano, Italy) that applied on the tip of the thin metallic blade a calibrated shock wave of 130 daN. The longitudinal movements imparted by the device promoted the penetration of the blade parallel to the long axis of the tooth (or each root) advancing apically in 2mm increments at both mesial and distal aspects with minimal hand pressure.

After applying the magnetoelectric device, each tooth/root could be easily removed without applying any latero-lateral force with luxators pushing in forward/rearward and upwards direction and with extraction forceps for residual roots exerting rotational force in a coronal direction.

Conventional tooth extraction

After clinical assessment of tooth to be extracted, periosteal elevators were used for reflecting the gingiva to expose the cemento-enamel junction and the extraction was carried out using conventional forceps and luxating elevators by dislodging the tooth without tooth sectioning, as per a simple extraction (that is, an intact tooth removal) without any mechanical device. No force other than manually was used to extract the tooth. Neither flaps were raised nor releasing incisions was performed.

Subsequently, for both groups a sterile re-absorbable gelatin sponge (Cutanplast® Dental, Dispotech S.r.l., Gordona (SO), Italy) was placed to fill the socket and secured with sutures. Sutures were used to stabilize collagen and blood clots.

Immediately after the surgery and domiciliary for oneweek, patients were asked to apply an oral amino-acids based gel with hyaluronic acid (Aminogam gel® of Polifarma Benessere S.r.l., Rome, Italy) after the oral hygiene procedures to reduce swelling and pain.

2.3. Outcomes

Descriptive variables were registered: age, gender, smoking habits, and tooth location.

Primary predictor variable

- test group "*ltr*", less traumatic tooth extraction; control group "*con*", conventional tooth extraction.
- Secondary predictor variable
- Tooth site: premolar versus molar; aspect: buccal versus palatal

Primary outcome variables

The measurer calculated anatomical variables based on volumetric and superficial features of the extraction site and expressed in cm^3/cm^2 to two decimal places. All anatomical measurements were positive.

V_{T0} and V_{T1}: volume of the alveolar ridge within the standardized VOI, respectively, at the intraoperative time point (T0) and 4 months after tooth extraction (T1) (Figure 2).

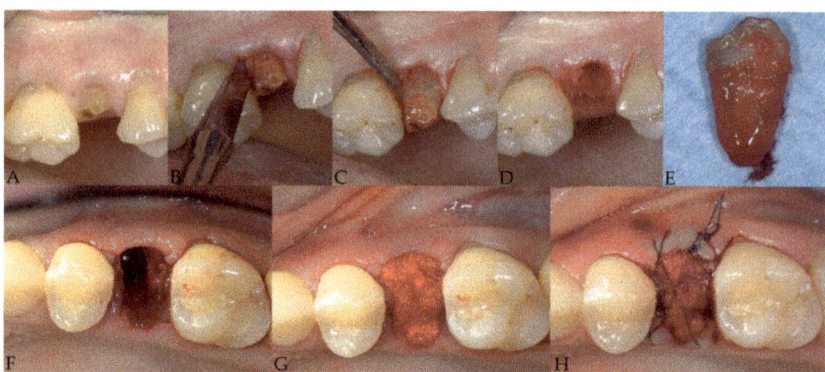

Figure 2. Clinical view of a less extraction technique. (**A**) preoperative; (**B**,**C**) electromagnetic tips for mesial and distal luxation; (**D**) extraction; (**E**) extracted tooth; (**F**) post extraction socket; (**G**) gelatin sponge; (**H**) sutures.

BS_{T0} and BS_{T1}: basal surface of the alveolar ridge or the area of the most apical axial) of the VOI box, respectively, at T0 and T1 (Figure 1).

Secondary outcome variables

All outcomes were obtained by a series of algebraic manipulations of the primary ones. The secondary outcomes were usually negative and represented a loss in volume or a reduction in surface.

Volume change of the alveolar ridge from T0 to T1, or ΔV (evaluated by subtracting the baseline value V_{T0} from that of the intraoperative survey V_{T1}) and its analogous in terms of percentage within the VOI, were respectively given by Equations (1) and (2):

$$\Delta V = V_{T1} - V_{T0} \tag{1}$$

$$\Delta V\% = 100 \cdot (V_{T1} - V_{T0})/V_{T0} \tag{2}$$

Change at basal surface with its loss in terms of percentage were given by Equations (3) and (4)

$$\Delta BS = BS_{T1} - BS_{T0} \tag{3}$$

$$\Delta BS\% = 100 \cdot (BS_{T1} - BS_{T0})/V_{T0} \tag{4}$$

2.4. Statistical Analysis

A statistician performed all analyses using a statistical tool from a Matrix Laboratory (Statistics Toolbox, MatLab 7.11; The MathWorks, Natick, MA, USA).

There was one extraction site per patient so that the two groups were independent; normal distribution for each outcome variable was checked, but not confirmed, by the Shapiro–Wilk test [29]. Moreover, the assumption of homoscedasticity for equality of variances was not met by Brown-Forsythe's test for all groups and subgroups investigated.

Wilcoxon tests were employed for pair-wise comparisons for matched and unmatched samples; Spearman's correlation assessed the strength of the bivariate association between the outcomes and the other variables.

The effects of the sample and the results of the power analysis were, respectively, determined with a power of 0.99, the reported sample size, and both measures of central tendency and dispersion.

The level of statistical significance was set at 0.01 for all analyses.

3. Results

In the present analysis, 48 patients were considered eligible. All the demographic data and variables' descriptions and dispersions about the extracted teeth ranked between the groups had been reported in Table 1. Healing following tooth extraction in 45 sites appeared uneventful; three sites showed swelling, redness, and flow of exudate resolved within one week of adjunctive antibiotic administration, as shown in Table 1.

Table 1. Demographic data and homogeneity analysis between the two groups, less traumatic tooth extraction (*ltr*) and conventional tooth extraction (*con*), with descriptive variables (gender male/female, Y/N, and bicuspids/molars ratio, Bd/Mr and swelling events Y/N). The assumption of homoscedasticity was not met by Brown-Forsythe's test for equality of variances F = 4.7130, df1 = 3, df2 = 92, p = 0.0042, and F = 4.6245, df1 = 3, df2 = 92, p = 0.0047 for overall volume variable and its buccal aspect. Bd, bicuspid; Mr, molar. Anatomical and outcome variables at baseline (T0) and at 4 months (T1, when the site was healed): volume of the alveolar ridge or V, basal surface or BS, and outcome variables (alveolar ridge volume and basal change percentages, respectively, ΔV% and BS%. Shapiro–Wilk test significance (p_{SW}); Wilcoxon rank-sum test significance between unpaired data (p_{Wu}); Wilcoxon signed-rank test significance between paired data (p_{Wp}); Results of Fischer test (p_F). Statistically-significant values are in bold. Report of calculated sample size (with power = 0.99) and calculated power.

Group	Less Traumatic Tooth Extraction (*ltr*)	Conventional Tooth Extraction (*con*)	p_F *ltr* vs. *con*
sample size	20	28	-
genders F/M	12/8	15/13	0.7710
Ratio Bd/Mr	8/12	9/19	0.7603
Smoke Y/N	2/18	2/26	1.0000
age (range)	53.4 ± 8.2 (41.0–70.0)	46.0 ± 10.9 (25.1–63.7)	-
swelling Y/N	1/19	2/26	1.0000

	primary predictor: experimental groups									
	N = 20		p_{Wp} times	N = 28		p_{Wp} times	p_{Wu} *ltr* vs. *con*		*ltr* vs. *con*	
Time X	T0	T1	T0 vs. T1	T0	T1	T0 vs. T1	T0	T1	sample size	power
V (cm^3)	1.22 ± 0.29	0.87 ± 0.34	**<0.0001**	1.22 ± 0.27	0.66 ± 0.19	**<0.0001**	0.9084	0.0346		
p_{SW} (SW)	0.2156	**0.0031**		0.4917	0.5950					
BS(cm^2)	1.47 ± 0.37	1.37 ± 0.38	**<0.0001**	1.59 ± 0.47	1.49 ± 0.49	**<0.0001**	0.4207	0.6157		
p_{SW} (SW)	0.3829	0.0983		0.5656	0.2511					
ΔV (cm^3)		−0.36 ± 0.12			−0.56 ± 0.11			**<0.0001**	17	1.00
p_{SW} (SW)		0.3050			0.3042					
ΔV%		−31.3 ± 13.3			−46.2 ± 5.8			**0.0001**	21	0.99
p_{SW} (SW)		0.0472			0.5962					
ΔBS(cm^2)		−0.10 ± 0.07			−0.10 ± 0.07			0.7458	N.D	0.00
p_{SW} (SW)		0.3581			0.3531					
ΔBS%		−6.8 ± 4.5			−7.2 ± 5.4			0.9583	7807	0.01
p_{SW} (SW)		0.0909			0.1936					

3.1. Primary Predictors: Procedures

The two groups were of similar sizes in terms of pristine surface area and baseline volume, while significant reductions of anatomical features were observed four months later in all the groups (Table 1 and Figure 3 with p-values ≤ 0.0002). In fact, in both groups, the volume losses (−0.36 ± 0.12 cm^3 and −0.56 ± 0.11 cm^3, respectively, for *ltr* and *con* group) and reduction of the basal surfaces (−0.10 ± 0.07 cm^2 for both of them) were registered at four-month follow-up, leading to a final alveolar ridge volume of 0.87 ± 0.34 cm^3 for less traumatic extractions and 0.66 ± 0.19 cm³ for conventional extractions. No significant differences were registered for outcomes related to the basal surface variables.

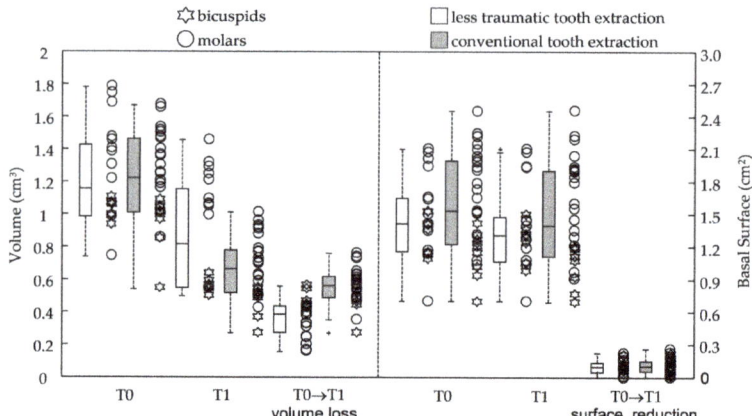

Figure 3. Scatter and box plots for the anatomical variables and outcomes at baseline (T0) and 4month postoperative time (T1) in *ltr* and *con* group; volumes V, basal surfaces BS, and their change at 3 months. In the box-and-whiskers plot, the box line represents the lower, median, and upper quartile values, the whisker lines include the rest of the data. Outliers (+) were data with values beyond the ends of the whiskers. Scatter data were ranked by tooth type.

Correlation analyses between each secondary outcome and all the anatomical variables were shown in Table 2. No significant correlations were reported for *ltr* group. In the conventional extraction group, the outcome related to volume resorption (ΔV) had a negative correlation with both the pristine volume (r_s −0.7588 with *p*-value < 0.0001), and basal surface at baseline (r_s −0.7122 with *p*-value < 0.0001).

Table 2. Spearman's correlation coefficients r_s with significances between outcome variables and overall anatomical variables for alveolar ridge modification in two groups, less traumatic tooth extraction (*ltr*) and conventional tooth extraction (*con*).

Outcome Variables	Procedure vs.	Less Traumatic Tooth Extraction (*ltr*)			Conventional Tooth Extraction (*con*)		
		V_{T0}	BS_{T0}	iH_{T0}	V_{T0}	BS_{T0}	iH_{T0}
ΔV	correlation coefficient (r_s)	0.3179	0.0188	0.4664	−0.7588	−0.7122	0.4412
	significance (two-tailed)	0.1720	0.9373	0.0313	**<0.0001**	**<0.0001**	0.0188
ΔBS	correlation coefficient (r_s)	0.1695	0.1061	0.1203	0.2436	0.2573	−0.3038
	significance (two-tailed)	0.4750	0.6562	0.6133	0.2115	0.1863	0.1160

3.2. Secondary Predictors: Tooth Aspect and Site

When extraction types were investigated for buccal or palatal/lingual aspects, the observed behaviors were similar to those recorded in the previous section and shown in Table 3; that is, significant differences had been recorded between *ltr* and *con* groups regarding the percentages of volume loss (with ranges from 28.6 to 34.4% and from 41.5 to 52.8%, respectively, for less traumatic and conventional procedure) with *p*-values ≤ 0.0046. Again, all the anatomical variables (V and BS) were significantly different between the two aspects (*p*-value ≤ 0.0004), but just the outcome ΔV% showed a higher rate in the conventional group when buccal (−52.8 ± 7.3%) and palatal aspect (−41.5 ± 8.4%) had been compared (*p*-value < 0.0001).

Table 3. Anatomical variables and outcomes for the group less traumatic tooth extraction (*ltr*) and conventional tooth extraction (*con*), at baseline (T0) and at 4 months (T1, when the site was healed) for the secondary predictor tooth aspect and location: buccal versus palatal and bicuspid versus molar. Volume of alveolar ridge or V, basal surface or BS, and outcome variables (percentages of Volume and Basal Surface change). Shapiro–Wilk test significance (p_{SW}); Wilcoxon rank-sum test significance between unpaired data (p_{Wu}); Wilcoxon signed-rank test significance between paired data (p_{Wp}). Statistically-significant values are in bold. Report of calculated sample size (with power = 0.99) and calculated power.

Group	Less Traumatic Tooth Extraction (*ltr*)			Conventional Tooth Extraction (*con*)			p_{Wu} *ltr* vs. *con*		*ltr* vs. *con*	
	N = 20		p_{Wp} Times	N = 28		p_{Wp} Times				
Time X	T0	T1	T0 vs. T1	T0	T1	T0 vs. T1	T0	T1	sample Size	power
				secondary predictor: buccal						
V (cm^3)	0.52 ± 0.15	0.35 ± 0.15	**<0.0001**	0.51 ± 0.14	0.24 ± 0.09	**<0.0001**	0.9084	**0.0196**		
p_{SW} (SW)	0.1979	**0.0434**		0.2889	0.2471					
BS(cm^2)	0.58 ± 0.14	0.53 ± 0.13	**0.0003**	0.65 ± 0.21	0.60 ± 0.21	**<0.0001**	0.2415	0.2499		
p_{SW} (SW)	0.9000	0.7803		0.1869	0.1184					
ΔV (cm^3)		−0.17 ± 0.05			−0.26 ± 0.07		**<0.0001**		24	0.97
p_{SW} (SW)		0.6222			0.1246					
ΔV%		−34.4 ± 13.1			−52.8 ± 7.3		**<0.0001**		150	0.22
p_{SW} (SW)		0.8268			0.8452					
ΔBS(cm^2)		−0.05 ± 0.04			−0.05 ± 0.04		0.6444		N.D	0.00
p_{SW} (SW)		0.1914			**0.0143**					
ΔBS%		−8.6 ± 6.7			−7.8 ± 6.4		0.6671		3268	0.01
p_{SW} (SW)		0.2789			**0.0456**					
				secondary predictor: palatal						
	N = 20		p_{Wp} times	N = 28		p_{Wp} times	p_{Wu} *ltr* vs. *con*		*ltr* vs. *con*	
Time X	T0	T1	T0 vs. T1	T0	T1	T0 vs. T1	T0	T1	sample size	power
V (cm^3)	0.71 ± 0.17	0.52 ± 0.19	**<0.0001**	0.71 ± 0.16	0.42 ± 0.13	**<0.0001**	0.9666	0.1549		
p_{SW} (SW)	0.0826	0.0598		0.1458	0.9979					
BS(cm^2)	0.89 ± 0.30	0.84 ± 0.32	**0.0002**	0.94 ± 0.29	0.89 ± 0.30	**<0.0001**	0.4771	0.6605		
p_{SW} (SW)	0.1706	0.0687		0.4612	0.2866					
ΔV (cm^3)		−0.20 ± 0.10			−0.29 ± 0.08		**0.0014**		48	0.72
p_{SW} (SW)		0.5916			0.3528					
ΔV%		−28.6 ± 15.1			−41.5 ± 8.4		**0.0046**		149	0.22
p_{SW} (SW)		**0.0289**			0.7460					
ΔBS(cm^2)		−0.04 ± 0.04			−0.06 ± 0.05		0.3270		261	0.11
p_{SW} (SW)		**0.0089**			**0.0129**					
ΔBS%		−5.6 ± 5.2			−6.7 ± 6.1		0.5203		1338	0.02
p_{SW} (SW)		**0.0021**			**0.0085**					
			p_{Wp} between buccal and palatal							
Time X	T0	T1		T0	T1					
V (cm^3)	**0.0003**	**0.0001**		**<0.0001**	**<0.0001**					
BS(cm^2)	**0.0002**	**0.0001**		**<0.0001**	**<0.0001**					
ΔV (cm^3)		0.3134			0.0855					
ΔV%		**0.0206**			**<0.0001**					
ΔBS(cm^2)		0.3812			0.2584					
ΔBS%		0.1024			0.6567					

Table 3. Cont.

Group	Less Traumatic Tooth Extraction (ltr)			Conventional Tooth Extraction (con)			p_{Wu} ltr vs. con		ltr vs. con	
	\multicolumn{3}{} secondary predictor: bicuspids								
	N = 8		p_{Wp} times	N = 9		p_{Wp} times				
Time X	T0	T1	T0 vs. T1	T0	T1	T0 vs. T1	T0	T1	sample size	power
V (cm³)	1.02 ± 0.06	0.56 ± 0.04	**0.0078**	0.95 ± 0.17	0.47 ± 0.09	**0.0039**	0.4650	**0.0058**		
p_{SW} (SW)	0.6037	0.3417		**0.0030**	**0.0090**					
BS(cm²)	1.33 ± 0.18	1.23 ± 0.18	**0.0078**	1.14 ± 0.22	1.03 ± 0.19	**0.0039**	0.1455	0.0879		
p_{SW} (SW)	0.1687	0.5479		0.5263	0.0577					
ΔV (cm³)		−0.46 ± 0.06			−0.47 ± 0.08			0.3203	2597	0.01
p_{SW} (SW)		0.2554			**0.0134**					
ΔV%		−44.9 ± 4.2			−50.0 ± 3.4			**0.0152**	29	0.51
p_{SW} (SW)		0.3197			0.3687					
ΔBS(cm²)		−0.10 ± 0.05			−0.11 ± 0.07			0.6058	1926	0.01
p_{SW} (SW)		0.2949			0.8733					
ΔBS%		−7.7 ± 3.5			−9.7 ± 5.8			0.4234	301	0.04
p_{SW} (SW)		0.8929			0.7720					
	\multicolumn{3}{} secondary predictor: molars								
	N = 12		p_{Wp} times	N = 19		p_{Wp} times	p_{Wu} ltr vs. con		ltr vs. con	
Time X	T0	T1	T0 vs. T1	T0	T1	T0 vs. T1	T0	T1	sample size	power
V (cm³)	1.37 ± 0.30	1.07 ± 0.28	**0.0005**	1.35 ± 0.21	0.75 ± 0.16	**0.0001**	0.7000	**0.0015**		
p_{SW} (SW)	0.5803	0.0831		0.6063	0.7979					
BS(cm²)	1.56 ± 0.43	1.47 ± 0.45	**0.0039**	1.80 ± 0.39	1.71 ± 0.42	**0.0003**	0.1618	0.2647		
p_{SW} (SW)	0.5858	0.4003		0.6182	0.6248					
ΔV (cm³)		−0.30 ± 0.10			−0.59 ± 0.10			**<0.0001**	6	1.00
p_{SW} (SW)		0.3988			0.3843					
ΔV%		−22.3 ± 8.4			−44.3 ± 5.8			**<0.0001**	5	1.00
p_{SW} (SW)		**0.0282**			0.6582					
ΔBS(cm²)		−0.09 ± 0.08			−0.10 ± 0.07			0.8233	2726	0.01
p_{SW} (SW)		0.2942			0.3087					
ΔBS%		−6.2 ± 5.2			−6.0 ± 4.9			0.9838	31268	0.01
p_{SW} (SW)		0.0934			0.1476					
	\multicolumn{3}{} p_{Wu} between bicuspids and molars								
Time X	T0	T1		T0	T1					
V (cm³)	**0.0096**	**0.0048**		**0.0004**	**0.0004**					
BS(cm²)	0.1425	0.2316		**0.0004**	**0.0004**					
ΔV (cm³)		**0.0010**			**0.0025**					
ΔV%		**0.0008**			**0.0063**					
ΔBS(cm²)		0.6712			0.4029					
ΔBS%		0.5118			0.1045					

When premolar and molar sites had been evaluated, the type of extraction showed a small impact on the volume loss; in fact, ΔVs and ΔV%s were, respectively, −0.46 ± 0.06 cm³ and −44.9 ± 4.2% for the less traumatic group and −0.47 ± 0.08 cm³ and −50.0 ± 3.4% for the conventional group without any significant differences.

However, when just molar tooth were considered, analysis of outcomes relating to the volume showed a better behavior in the less traumatic procedure (ΔV = −0.30 ± 0.10 cm³ and ΔV% = −22.3 ± 8.4%) when compared to the conventional extractions (ΔV = −0.59 ± 0.10 cm³ and ΔV% = −44.3 ± 5.8%) with p-values < 0.0001.

4. Discussion

The purpose of this retrospective control study was to test the effectiveness of posterior single tooth extraction with or without a less traumatic extraction procedure in preserving existing alveolar ridge contours of the fresh socket using an intraoral laser scanner. Intraoperative digital cast model was compared to that of the healed site obtained four months after tooth extraction, before rehabilitation with implant-supported fixed single crown prosthesis. The stereolithographic files were voxelized and digitally superimposed by a matrix laboratory. Detailed analyses of contour modifications were performed on two fused voxelized .stl clouds.

It was often difficult to precisely define the meaning of an "atraumatic extraction" when considering the wide variety of described extraction techniques. As said, nevertheless, most of described atraumatic procedures with or without the use of several and special tools could certainly cause less damage to the tissues surrounding teeth, but, to a certain degree, still traumatized the bone to some extent [7,30].

So, all the other conventional or experimental extracting procedures, according to this view, could be defined as traumatic or less-traumatic ones. There was no question that any force application in horizontal directions could affect, in single-rooted teeth, alveolar bone remodeling more than rotational movements, so the application of forces in the buccal/palatal directions was much worse than those in the mesial/distal directions [31].

The final point needed to describe a less traumatic extraction technique was the use of any device whose primary function was breaking of periodontal fibers and removing conical roots without overexpansion of the alveolar socket.

The energy translated by the magnetoelectrical device into pulse pressure, which moved the subluxating periotome blade applied a vertical compressive and penetrating force along the root length detached the root from the surrounding alveolar tissues, and left intact the bony plate. Once each root was subluxated, it could be pulled out by using forceps for residual extraction of dental roots in a simple rotational movement [12].

Surgical sectioning was required when it appeared necessary to convert a posterior tooth into a multiple "single-rooted" one. On the contrary, in the event of fused or convergent roots, a multiple rooted tooth could be removed without sectioning [23].

The present study suggested that alveolar ridges of less traumatic extraction group reported at the four-month survey significantly (p-value = 0.0001) lower volume loss (31.3%) versus those treated with conventional traumatic extraction procedures with forceps and luxators (46.2%). This was true for both the aspects (buccal and lingual/palatal), even if just for volumetric outcomes. In the present study, non-significant dimensional changes were observed in the basal surface, with a small reduction registered in the volume of interest (decrease ranging from 5.6 and 8.6%). This was in line with evidence-based information reported in the literature on the factors affecting ridge width and height modification after tooth removal such as a flap or flapless technique, smoking habit, drugs administration during healing, number and shape of roots, and the status of the buccal bony plate (thin or fenestrated) [14,32,33].

Results regarding the behavior of alveolar bone remodeling in posterior areas were scanty. However, some studies attested that naturally healing sites that underwent tooth extraction showed a loss in height ranging from 1.4 to 3.6 mm and a reduction in width ranging from 2.3 to 4.5 mm irrespective of tooth site [34–37]. Some studies suggested that ridge preservation using low resorbing xenograft could considerably limit the amount of horizontal ridge resorption when compared with tooth extraction alone: a difference ranged between the two groups from -3.33 to -2 mm [19,38]. However, no information was provided regarding the type of extraction (more or less traumatic). When changes in the volume of the post-extraction sites underwent no socket ridge preservation were investigated, Sbordone and co-workers found that ridge preservation compensated for the postextraction alveolar ridge resorption with a loss of about 22% in the external contour [16]. Whereas, when clinicians left the extraction socket undisturbed, this might result in an alveolar contour shrinkage close to 40% after three to four months [16]. However, a less traumatic tooth extraction could counteract a volume loss of 10% leading to a volume loss of −31.3% as reported in the present findings. Moreover, when subgroups related to the tooth site were analyzed separately, molars of the less traumatic group suffered a significantly smaller loss in terms of volume outcomes (22.3%) than that of the traumatic extractions (44.3%). This did not happen in the bicuspid areas. Tooth type (bicuspids versus molars) seemed to influence the magnitude of the three-dimensional (3D) shape changes when less traumatic extraction had been performed in the posterior areas.

In this view, tooth extraction without damaging the hard and soft tissues of the post extractive socket was just the first step. Some authors suggested that the preservation of the socket volume was dependent first and foremost on maintaining pristine volume during extraction and then on clothing the socket to prevent contact between the healing tissues and the intraoral environment. This could be achieved not by filling the post-extraction socket with slow resorbing materials, but rather by using a tooth-like emergence profile when an immediate implant had been placed or by using an immediate pontic (very similar to the emergence profile of the natural tooth). With advances in three-dimensional printing, the use of materials as biocompatible as possible had offered new clinical opportunities. These new techniques could be used to produce scaffold for tissues' reconstruction with a highly precise and accurate design [39] or to fabricate any structure of mechanical interest in dentistry, which appeared to be individualized for each patient (for example surgical guides and orthodontic power-arms) [40,41].

The limitations of the present study might be an error generated during the acquisition of the arch digital impression. The presence of blood and spit during the production of the digital cast could be a primary source of the inaccuracy of the present optical scanning technique. No extrapolation could be made as to whether the volume resorption was caused by loss of soft tissue or underlying bone. Finally, the small number of patients/casts in each group might be another bias that could affect the measurement of true effectiveness, in terms of the percentages of loss of the external contours.

The use of a magnetoelectrical device probably minimized mechanical impacts on the alveolar tissues resulting in a reduction in volume two times that of sites with more traumatic tooth extraction, as the combined result of teeth segmentation and roots subluxation. In comparison with other conventional techniques for less traumatic tooth extraction, the magnetoelectric device played the same role as the periotomes, but with an additional feature of mesial/distal subluxation. Moreover, an advantage when using the magnetoelectric devices was that the instrument produced less heat and requires less cooling than the conventional rotary cutting, sonosurgery, piezosurgery, and piezoelectric devices [42,43].

However, it might be said that the present study included teeth with no buccal or palatal/lingual bone defects involving the alveolar crest. Thus, it is important to note that the applicability and results of the present procedure are not directly extensible to such severely damaged alveolar sockets.

5. Conclusions

The four-month analysis test group showed a reduced loss of the external contour when compared to the conventional tooth extraction technique. However, the less traumatic procedures seemed to be able to better preserve the volume of the alveolar crest (reduction close to 22% with less traumatic extraction) even if just for molars.

Tooth position (bicuspids versus molars) seemed to affect volume loss but not shrinkage of the basal surface with the molar site generally favored in volume preservation.

Author Contributions: Conceptualization, G.B.M.-F. and U.C.; Methodology, U.C.; Software, P.T.; Validation, R.C. and G.C.; Formal analysis, P.T.; Investigation, R.C. and G.C.; Resources, S.C. and U.C.; Data curation, G.C. and P.T.; Writing—original draft preparation, S.C. and P.T.; Writing—review and editing, P.T. and R.C.; Visualization, G.B.M.-F.; Supervision, P.T.; Project administration, G.B.M.-F. and U.C.; Funding acquisition, U.C. All authors have read and agreed to the published version of the manuscript.

Funding: This research received no external funding.

Institutional Review Board Statement: The study was conducted according to the guidelines of the Declaration of Helsinki of 2008 and updated in 2013 and was approved by the local Ethics Committee (Ethics Committee 2626–2008, PROT No. 58183 of the University of Pisa. Each patient agreed to participate in the study filling in a written informed consent.

Informed Consent Statement: Written informed consent was obtained from all subjects involved in the study.

Data Availability Statement: Additional data may be available if requested to the institute.

Conflicts of Interest: The authors declare no conflict of interest.

Abbreviations

LTETs	Less Traumatic Extraction Techniques
.stl	stereolithographic
VOI	Volume Of Interest
V	Volume of alveolar ridge
BS	Basal Surface
ltr	less traumatic tooth extraction group
con	conventional tooth extraction group

Appendix A

```
[x, y, z, c] = stlread('FILENAME OF THE STL');
% voxel dimension (Paolo Toti April 2019)
Dvox = 0.3
Sz = size(c); meshXYZ = zeros(Sz(2),3,3);
xx = reshape(x,3*Sz(2),1); Xmin = min(xx); Xmax = max(xx);
yy = reshape(y,3*Sz(2),1); Ymin = min(yy); Ymax = max(yy);
zz = reshape(z,3*Sz(2),1); Zmin = min(zz); Zmax = max(zz);
Dim = [XminXmaxZminZmaxYminYmax];
x1 = (x − Xmin)/Dvox; y1 = (y − Ymin)/Dvox; z1 = (z − Zmin)/Dvox;
xx1 = reshape(x1,3*Sz(2),1); yy1 = reshape(y1,3*Sz(2),1); zz1 = reshape(z1,3*Sz(2),1);
dimx = round(max(xx1)); dimy = round(max(yy1)); dimz = round(max(zz1));
for i = 1:Sz(2)
meshXYZ(i,:,:) = [x1(:,i)';y1(:,i)';z1(:,i)'];
end
[faces,vertices] = CONVERT_meshformat(meshXYZ);
FV1 = struct('vertices',vertices,'faces',faces);
J1 = polygon2voxel(FV1,[dimx, dimy, dimz],'none'); J2 = imfill(J1,'holes'); patch(x,y,z,c)
patch(isosurface(J2,0.8),'facecolor',[0 0 1],'edgecolor','none', camlight;view(3)
axis([0dimx0 dimy 0dimz ])
fileCount = 1; sequenceStartNo = 1; sequenceEndNo = dimy; finalZsectional = round(dimy/2);
path2 = 'FINAL PATH FOR DCM'
path3 = 'METAFILE PATH FOR DCM'
basename = 'IM'; fileExtension = '.dcm'; Nmin = sequenceStartNo; Nmax = sequenceEndNo;
D001 = zeros(280,280,sequenceEndNo); DFT = size(J2)
for i = 1:dimz
dh = DFT(1); dj = DFT(2);
for h = 1:dh;
for j = 1:dj;
D001(h,j,i) = J2(h,j,i);
end
end
end
imagesc(D001(:,:,int8(dimz./2)),[0 1]); colormap(gray);
```

```
for i = sequenceStartNo:sequenceEndNo
if i< 10
sequenceNo = strcat('000',num2str(i));
elseif ((10 <= i ) & (i< 100))
sequenceNo = strcat('00',num2str(i));
elseif ((100 <= i ) & (i<1000))
sequenceNo = strcat('0',num2str(i));
elseif 1000 <i
error('More than 1000 files selected')
end
filename2 = strcat(path2,basename,sequenceNo,'.dcm');
filename3 = strcat(path3,basename,sequenceNo,fileExtension);
metadata = dicominfo(filename3);
D002 = D001.*2000; D003(:,:,i) = imrotate(D002(:,:,i),0,'bilinear','crop'); X017(:,:,i) = int16(D003(:,:,i) − 1);
dicomwrite(X017(:,:,i),filename2, metadata)
if fileCount == 1
dicomHeaderInfo = dicominfo(filename3)
isotropicVoxelDimension = dicomHeaderInfo.PixelSpacing(1);
end
fileCount = fileCount + 1;
end
```

Appendix B

```
% ssA, ssB, ssC ... are data matrices at the different time points
threshold = 1000
ppA = ones(280,280,sequenceEndNo);
for i = 1:sequenceEndNo
d = 280; for h = 1:d; for j = 1:d;
if ssA(h,j,i) > threshold
ppA(h,j,i) = ssA(h,j,i);
end
end
end
end
```

References

1. Schropp, L.; Wenzel, A.; Kostopoulos, L.; Karring, T. Bone healing and soft tissue contour changes following single-tooth extraction: A clinical and radiographic 12-month prospective study. *Int. J. Periodontics Restor. Dent.* **2003**, *23*, 313–323.
2. Van derWeijden, F.; Dell'Acqua, F.; Slot, D.E. Alveolar bone dimensional changes of post-extraction sockets in humans: A systematic review. *J. Clin. Periodontol.* **2009**, *36*, 1048–1058. [CrossRef] [PubMed]
3. Marconcini, S.; Denaro, M.; Cosola, S.; Gabriele, M.; Toti, P.; Mijiritsky, E.; Proietti, A.; Basolo, F.; Giammarinaro, E.; Covani, U. Myofibroblast Gene Expression Profile after Tooth Extraction in the Rabbit. *Materials* **2019**, *12*, 3697. [CrossRef] [PubMed]
4. Chen, S.T.; Wilson, T.G., Jr.; Hämmerle, C.H. Immediate or early placement of implants following tooth extraction: Review of biologic basis, clinical procedures, and outcomes. *Int. J. Oral Maxillofac. Implant.* **2004**, *19*, 12–25.
5. De Santis, D.; Sinigaglia, S.; Pancera, P.; Faccioni, P.; Portelli, M.; Luciano, U.; Cosola, S.; Penarrocha, D.; Bertossi, D.; Nocini, R.; et al. An overview of socket preservation. *J. Biol. Regul. Homeost. Agents* **2019**, *33* (Suppl. 1), 55–59.
6. Ten Heggeler, J.M.; Slot, D.E.; Van der Weijden, G.A. Effect of socket preservation therapies following tooth extraction in non-molar regions in humans: A systematic review. *Clin. Oral Implant. Res.* **2011**, *22*, 779–788. [CrossRef]
7. Oghli, A.A.; Steveling, H. Ridge preservation following tooth extraction: A comparison between atraumatic extraction and socket seal surgery. *Quintessence Int.* **2010**, *41*, 605–609.
8. Avila-Ortiz, G.; Elangovan, S.; Kramer, K.W.; Blanchette, D.; Dawson, D.V. Effect of alveolar ridge preservation after tooth extraction: A systematic review and meta-analysis. *J. Dent. Res.* **2014**, *93*, 950–958. [CrossRef]
9. Quayle, A.A. Atraumatic removal of teeth and root fragments in dental implantology. *Int. J. Oral Maxillofac. Implant.* **1990**, *5*, 293–296.
10. Babbush, C.A. A new atraumatic system for tooth removal and immediate implant restoration. *Implant Dent.* **2007**, *16*, 139–145. [CrossRef]

11. Dym, H.; Weiss, A. Exodontia: Tips and techniques for better outcomes. *Dent. Clin.* **2012**, *56*, 245–266. [CrossRef]
12. Hämmerle, C.H.; Chen, S.T.; Wilson, T.G., Jr. Consensus statements and recommended clinical procedures regarding the placement of implants in extraction sockets. *Int. J. Oral Maxillofac. Implant.* **2004**, *19*, 26–28.
13. Niemiec, B.A. Extraction techniques. *Top. Companion Anim. Med.* **2008**, *23*, 97–105. [CrossRef] [PubMed]
14. Leblebicioglu, B.; Hegde, R.; Yildiz, V.O.; Tatakis, D.N. Immediate effects of tooth extraction on ridge integrity and dimensions. *Clin. Oral Investig.* **2015**, *19*, 1777–1784. [CrossRef] [PubMed]
15. Fabrizio, F.; Grusovin, M.G.; Gavatta, M.; Vercellotti, T. Clinical efficacy of a new fully piezoelectric technique for third molar root extraction without using manual tools: A clinical randomized controlled study. *Quintessence Int.* **2020**, *51*, 406–414. [CrossRef]
16. Sbordone, C.; Toti, P.; Martuscelli, R.; Guidetti, F.; Porzio, M.; Sbordone, L. Evaluation of volumetric dimensional changes in posterior extraction sites with and without ARP using a novel imaging device. *Clin. Implant Dent. Relat. Res.* **2017**, *19*, 1044–1053. [CrossRef] [PubMed]
17. Vanhoutte, V.; Rompen, E.; Lecloux, G.; Rues, S.; Schmitter, M.; Lambert, F. A methodological approach to assessing alveolar ridge preservation procedures in humans: Soft tissue profile. *Clin. Oral Implant. Res.* **2014**, *25*, 304–309. [CrossRef]
18. Coomes, A.M.; Mealey, B.L.; Huynh-Ba, G.; Barboza-Arguello, C.; Moore, W.S.; Cochran, D.L. Buccal bone formation after flapless extraction: A randomized, controlled clinical trial comparing recombinant human bone morphogenetic protein 2/absorbable collagen carrier and collagen sponge alone. *J. Periodontol.* **2014**, *85*, 525–535. [CrossRef]
19. Cardaropoli, D.; Tamagnone, L.; Roffredo, A.; Gaveglio, L. Relationship between the buccal bone plate thickness and the healing of postextraction sockets with/without ridge preservation. *Int. J. Periodontics Restor. Dent.* **2014**, *34*, 211–217. [CrossRef]
20. Walker, C.J.; Prihoda, T.J.; Mealey, B.L.; Lasho, D.J.; Noujeim, M.; Huynh-Ba, G. Evaluation of Healing at Molar Extraction Sites With and Without Ridge Preservation: A Randomized Controlled Clinical Trial. *J. Periodontol.* **2017**, *88*, 241–249. [CrossRef]
21. Saund, D.; Dietrich, T. Minimally-invasive tooth extraction: Doorknobs and strings revisited! *Dent. Updat.* **2013**, *40*, 325–326. [CrossRef]
22. Crespi, R.; Cappare, P.; Gherlone, E.F. Electrical mallet in implants placed in fresh extraction sockets with simultaneous osteotome sinus floor elevation. *Int. J. Oral Maxillofac. Implant.* **2013**, *28*, 869–874. [CrossRef] [PubMed]
23. Crespi, R.; Bruschi, G.B.; Capparé, P.; Gherlone, E. The utility of the electric mallet. *J. Craniofac. Surg.* **2014**, *25*, 793–795. [CrossRef]
24. Michelinakis, G.; Apostolakis, D.; Kamposiora, P.; Papavasiliou, G.; Özcan, M. The direct digital workflow in fixed implant prosthodontics: A narrative review. *BMC Oral Health* **2021**, *21*, 37. [CrossRef] [PubMed]
25. Siqueira, R.; Galli, M.; Chen, Z.; Mendonça, G.; Meirelles, L.; Wang, H.L.; Chan, H.L. Intraoral scanning reduces procedure time and improves patient comfort in fixed prosthodontics and implant dentistry: A systematic review. *Clin. Oral Investig.* **2021**, *25*, 6517–6531. [CrossRef] [PubMed]
26. Barone, A.; Toti, P.; Menchini-Fabris, G.B.; Derchi, G.; Marconcini, S.; Covani, U. Extra oral digital scanning and imaging superimposition for volume analysis of bone remodeling after tooth extraction with and without 2 types of particulate porcine mineral insertion: A randomized controlled trial. *Clin. Implant Dent. Relat. Res.* **2017**, *19*, 750–759. [CrossRef]
27. Menchini-Fabris, G.B.; Toti, P.; Crespi, G.; Covani, U.; Furlotti, L.; Crespi, R. Effect of Different Timings of Implant Insertion on the Bone Remodeling Volume around Patients' Maxillary Single Implants: A 2–3 Years Follow-Up. *Int. J. Environ. Res. Public Health* **2020**, *17*, 6790. [CrossRef] [PubMed]
28. Crespi, R.; Fabris, G.B.M.; Crespi, G.; Toti, P.; Marconcini, S.; Covani, U. Effects of different loading protocols on the bone remodeling volume of immediate maxillary single implants: A 2- to 3-year follow-up. *Int. J. Oral Maxillofac. Implant.* **2019**, *34*, 953–962. [CrossRef]
29. Herrmann, I.; Lekholm, U.; Holm, S.; Kultje, C. Evaluation of patient and implant characteristics as potential prognostic factors for oral implant failures. *Int. J. Oral Maxillofac. Implant.* **2005**, *20*, 220–230.
30. Regev, E.; Lustmann, J.; Nashef, R. Atraumatic teeth extraction in bisphosphonate-treated patients. *J. Oral Maxillofac. Surg.* **2008**, *66*, 1157–1161. [CrossRef]
31. Muska, E.; Walter, C.; Knight, A.; Taneja, P.; Bulsara, Y.; Hahn, M.; Desai, M.; Dietrich, T. Atraumatic vertical tooth extraction: A proof of principle clinical study of a novel system. *Oral Surg. Oral Med. Oral Pathol. Oral Radiol.* **2013**, *116*, 303–310. [CrossRef] [PubMed]
32. Nevins, M.; Camelo, M.; De Paoli, S.; Friedland, B.; Schenk, R.K.; Parma-Benfenati, S.; Simion, M.; Tinti, C.; Wagenberg, B. A study of the fate of the buccal wall of extraction sockets of teeth with prominent roots. *Int. J. Periodontics Restor. Dent.* **2006**, *26*, 19–29. [CrossRef]
33. Moya-Villaescusa, M.J.; Sánchez-Pérez, A. Measurement of ridge alterations following tooth removal: A radiographic study in humans. *Clin. Oral Implant. Res.* **2010**, *21*, 237–242. [CrossRef] [PubMed]
34. Barone, A.; Aldini, N.N.; Fini, M.; Giardino, R.; Calvo Guirado, J.L.; Covani, U. Xenograft versus extraction alone for ridge preservation after tooth removal: A clinical and histomorphometric study. *J. Periodontol.* **2008**, *79*, 1370–1377. [CrossRef]
35. Araújo, M.G.; da Silva, J.C.C.; de Mendonça, A.F.; Lindhe, J. Ridge alterations following grafting of fresh extraction sockets in man. A randomized clinical trial. *Clin. Oral Implant. Res.* **2015**, *26*, 407–412. [CrossRef] [PubMed]
36. Jambhekar, S.; Kernen, F.; Bidra, A.S. Clinical and histologic outcomes of socket grafting after flapless tooth extraction: A systematic review of randomized controlled clinical trials. *J. Prosthet. Dent.* **2015**, *113*, 371–382. [CrossRef]

37. Iorio-Siciliano, V.; Ramaglia, L.; Blasi, A.; Bucci, P.; Nuzzolo, P.; Riccitiello, F.; Nicolò, M. Dimensional changes following alveolar ridge preservation in the posterior area using bovine-derived xenografts and collagen membrane compared to spontaneous healing: A 6-month randomized controlled clinical trial. *Clin. Oral Investig.* **2020**, *24*, 1013–1023. [CrossRef]
38. Barone, A.; Ricci, M.; Tonelli, P.; Santini, S.; Covani, U. Tissue changes of extraction sockets in humans: A comparison of spontaneous healing vs. ridge preservation with secondary soft tissue healing. *Clin. Oral Implant. Res.* **2013**, *24*, 1231–1237. [CrossRef]
39. Tellisi, N.; Ashammakhi, N.A.; Billi, F.; Kaarela, O. Three Dimensional Printed Bone Implants in the Clinic. *J. Craniofac. Surg.* **2018**, *29*, 2363–2367. [CrossRef]
40. Wegmüller, L.; Halbeisen, F.; Sharma, N.; Kühl, S.; Thieringer, F.M. Consumer vs. High-End 3D Printers for Guided Implant Surgery—An In Vitro Accuracy Assessment Study of Different 3D Printing Technologies. *J. Clin. Med.* **2021**, *10*, 4894. [CrossRef]
41. Thurzo, A.; Kociš, F.; Novák, B.; Czako, L.; Varga, I. Three-Dimensional Modeling and 3D Printing of Biocompatible Orthodontic Power-Arm Design with Clinical Application. *Appl. Sci.* **2021**, *11*, 9693. [CrossRef]
42. Heinemann, F.; Hasan, I.; Kunert-Keil, C.; Götz, W.; Gedrange, T.; Spassov, A.; Schweppe, J.; Gredes, T. Experimental and histological investigations of the bone using two different oscillating osteotomy techniques compared with conventional rotary osteotomy. *Ann. Anat.* **2012**, *194*, 165–170. [CrossRef] [PubMed]
43. Papadimitriou, D.E.; Geminiani, A.; Zahavi, T.; Ercoli, C. Sonosurgery for atraumatic tooth extraction: A clinical report. *J. Prosthet. Dent.* **2012**, *108*, 339–343. [CrossRef]

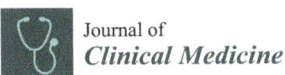

Article

Trueness of Intraoral Scanners in Implant-Supported Rehabilitations: An In Vitro Analysis on the Effect of Operators' Experience and Implant Number

Paolo Pesce [1,*], Francesco Bagnasco [2], Nicolò Pancini [2], Marco Colombo [3], Luigi Canullo [4], Francesco Pera [5], Eriberto Bressan [6], Marco Annunziata [7] and Maria Menini [2]

1 Department of Surgical Sciences (DISC), University of Genoa, Ospedale S. Martino, L. Rosanna Benzi 10, 16132 Genoa, Italy
2 Department of Surgical Sciences (DISC), Division of Prosthodontics, University of Genoa, Ospedale S. Martino, L. Rosanna Benzi 10, 16132 Genoa, Italy; fcbagna5@hotmail.it (F.B.); pancini.91@gmail.com (N.P.); maria.menini@unige.it (M.M.)
3 Private Practice, 20100 Milan, Italy; m.colombo.dds@gmail.com
4 Department of Periodontology, University of Bern, 3012 Bern, Switzerland; luigicanullo@yahoo.com
5 CIR Dental School, Department of Surgical Sciences, University of Turin, 10126 Turin, Italy; francesco.pera@unito.it
6 Department of Periodontology, Dental Clinic, School of Dentistry, University of Padova, 35122 Padova, Italy; eriberto.bressan@unipd.it
7 Multidisciplinary Department of Medical-Surgical and Dental Specialties, University of Campania "Luigi Vanvitelli", 81100 Naples, Italy; marco.annunziata@unicampania.it
* Correspondence: paolo.pesce@unige.it

Abstract: (1) Background: Intraoral scanners (IOS) are widely used in prosthodontics. However, a good trueness is mandatory to achieve optimal clinical results. The aim of the present in vitro study was to compare two IOS considering the operator's experience and different implant clinical scenarios. (2) Methods: Two IOS (IT—Itero, Align Technology; and OP—Opera MC, Opera System, Monaco) were compared simulating three different clinical scenarios: single implant, two implants, and full-arch rehabilitation. Ten scans were taken for each configuration by two different operators (one expert, one inexperienced); influence of operator experience and the type of scanner used was investigated. (3) Results: Trueness of the scans differed between the experienced and non-experienced operator and this difference was statistically significant in all the three scenarios ($p = 0.000$–0.001, 0.037). A significant difference was present between the scanners ($p = 0.000$), in the two-implant and full-arch scenarios ($p = 0.00$). (4) Conclusions: Experience of the operator significantly affect trueness of IT and OP scanners. A statistically significant difference was present among IOS in the two-implant and full-arch scenarios.

Keywords: dental implants; digital impression; intraoral scanner

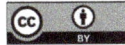

1. Introduction

Precision and accuracy of the impression is mandatory to achieve satisfactory clinical outcomes in implant prosthodontics and different materials and techniques have been proposed to reduce possible errors during the step of data transfer to the dental laboratory [1]. In particular, over the last two decades, digital impression spread in clinical practice, in parallel with the development of computer-aided design and manufacturing (CAD/CAM), contributing to the increasingly popular digitalization of the prosthodontic workflow.

Multiple methods have been proposed to collect three-dimensional data of teeth and implants through optical cameras and laser scans [2] and numerous research have been conducted to demonstrate the reliability of these technologies.

As opposed to traditional impression, digital impressions taken with intra oral scanners (IOS) is well tolerated by the patient, since it does not require the use of conventional materials and is technically simpler for the professional [3].

Additionally, thanks to IOS the quality of the impression can be immediately verified analyzing virtual models on the computer, without producing a physical model [4]. This allows for saving time and space necessary for storing analogic models, and impressions can be sent to the dental laboratory by e-mail, eliminating shipping time and costs. Last but not least, the clinician can profit of a more effective communication with the patient together with a powerful marketing tool.

Several studies have reported high levels of accuracy and precision of IOS, both in vitro and in vivo [3,5–9].

Ender et al. defined the trueness as the comparison between a control STL dataset and a test STL dataset and reported that, in the case of a partial scan, the average trueness of IOS technologies is between 20 and 48 μm and the accuracy is between 4 and 16 μm compared to conventional impression, concluding that current scanners are clinically suitable for common practice [10–12].

On the contrary, Keul et al. compared the accuracy of five intraoral scanners to indirect digitalization using laboratory scanners and reported that direct digitalization was not superior to the indirect method [13].

A recent in vitro study analyzed the performance of two different IOS considering the operator experience. The results showed that scans of single implant rehabilitations or bridges with two pontic elements display a very high level of accuracy, in contrast with full-arch rehabilitations that presented the worst trueness [8].

The aim of the present in vitro study was to evaluate the trueness of a new recently commercialized IOS (OP—Opera MC, Opera System, Monaco) comparing it with one of the most used IOS actually available on the market (IT—Itero, Align Technology), comparing different clinical scenarios and the outcomes of operators with different clinical experience.

The null hypothesis tested was that no differences existed in trueness of intraoral scans made using different IOS, by clinicians with different learning curve and in case of different implant number.

2. Materials and Methods

In the present in vitro investigation, the same methodology was applied as reported in a previously published study [8]. Three plaster master casts were made reproducing three different implant clinical situations (Figure 1):

1. Single implant in zone 16;
2. Two implants with two pontic elements (zone 13–16);
3. Full-arch rehabilitation with 4 implants (zone 13–16–23–26).

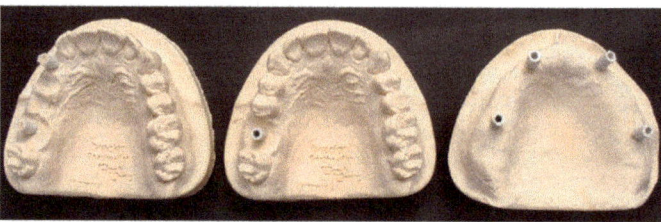

Figure 1. Images of the plaster models.

The master casts were the same used in the previously published study [8]. Scanbodies (A-INT-CAMTRA330, Sweden & Martina, Padua, Italy) were screwed on each implant analogue reproducing a 3.30 mm Prama implant (A-ANABU-330, Sweden & Martina, Padua, Italy).

The two operators scanning the master casts were a clinician experienced with IOS (more than two years of experience with digital impression systems) and an inexperienced clinician who had never used an IOS before.

The two operators performed 10 scans for each plaster model, using the OS and the IT (total of 60 scans performed).

The "S" scan path has been applied for each scan and scanner; the tip followed the entire arch with a fluid movement starting from the last tooth of the first quadrant to the contralateral tooth while zig-zagging from vestibular to palatal and back.

To test the trueness of the scans, the three models were scanned with a reference laboratory scanner (ScanRider, V-GER) with a standard resolution of 25 to 50 µm, an average error (accuracy) of 5 to 10 µm, and a precision (standard deviation [SD]) of 15 to 30 µm. The digital impressions were then imported into a reverse engineering software (Geomagic Studio 2012, 3D Systems, Morrisville, NC, USA) and superimposed on the reference dataset. The superimposition consisted of two different procedures:

1. First, the 3-point recording function was used, where three reference points were identified on the surface of the scanbodies. This function made it possible to compare a first approximate alignment of the two models (scan deriving from the operator and reference scan) using three-dimensional (3D) surfaces.
2. The aligned models were then subjected to a cutting process with the aim of standardizing the dimensions of the different scans relative to the areas of interest around the scanbodies. A different shear pattern was used for each clinical scenario.
3. Subsequently, the best-fit algorithm was applied for the final superimposition and recording of discrepancies. With this second alignment step, after defining the reference data and parameters for registration, the polygons forming the selected models were automatically overlapped. For this final recording, a Refined Iterative Closest Point (RICP) algorithm was used, and discrepancies between the reference data and those deriving from the overlapping models were minimized using a point-to-plane method, calculating the congruence between corresponding specific structures. The same alignment parameters were used for all overlapping procedures: 100 maximum interactions and sample size set to 1000 triangles.

Distances between the corresponding reference areas and all overlapping models were color-coded using the 3D deviation function (Figure 2). Then, mean values and standard deviations were calculated.

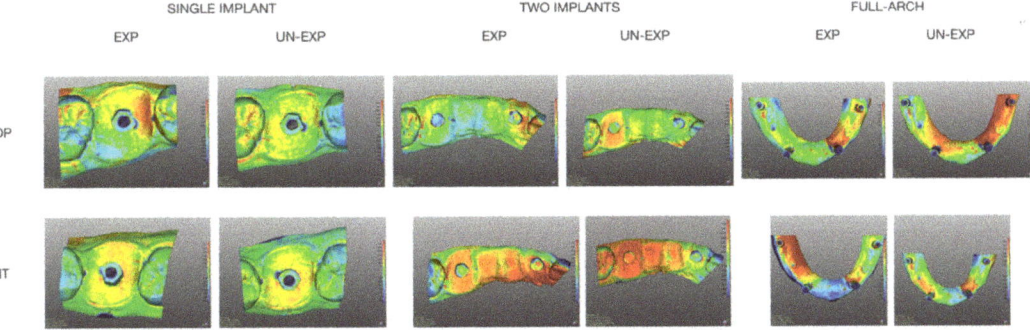

Figure 2. Evaluation of average deviation between RD (reference dataset) and DI (digital impression). Distances were color-coded using the 3D deviation function. IT (Itero IOS); OP (Opera system); EXP (expert operator) UN-EXP (unexperienced operator).

Statistical analyses were performed with SPSS (IBM SPSS Statistics for iOS, Version 25.0. IBM Corp, Armonk, NY, USA) software.

Measurements obtained were divided into three samples based on the different clinical scenario (single implant, two implants, full-arch).

For each group, a comparison was made between the data obtained from each scanner using the non-parametric Mann–Whitney test (U-test) for two independent groups.

Subsequently, for each clinical scenario analyzed, the weight of the various independent variables analyzed (scanner, expert or un-expert operator) were analyzed with a multivariate factor analysis.

3. Results

Mean values of trueness comparing data deriving from the scans are reported in Table 1.

Table 1. Trueness (mean (SD)), in μm. Trueness decrease in the full-arch scenario (OP opera system; IT Itero IOS).

Operator	Single Implant		Two Implants		Full-Arch	
	OP	IT	OP	IT	OP	IT
Experienced	8.62 (2.13)	8.45 (1.62)	5.56 (2.29)	18.29 (3.19)	66.23 (17.53)	96.02 (12.05)
Un-experienced	10.9 (2.06)	12.59 (2.19)	7.81 (1.70)	22.01 (2.32)	39.82 (7.18)	140.84 (13.97)
p Mann–Whitney (scanner)	0.417		0.000		0.000	
p Multivariate factor analysis (operator experience)	0.000		0.001		0.037	
p Multivariate factor analysis (scanner)	0.269		0.000		0.000	
p Multivariate factor analysis (scanner and operator experience)	0.153		0.381		0.000	

The statistical analysis revealed that the choice of the scanner was significant ($p < 0.05$) only in clinical scenarios with two implants and in full-arches (Mann–Whitney U-test).

The experience of the operator who performs the scans, on the other hand, was always significant in all the three clinical scenarios evaluated. If, on the other hand, the choice of the scanner and the experience of the operator were considered simultaneously, they were only significant in cases of full-arch.

4. Discussion

Currently, digital impression is widespread in implant dentistry; however, clinical outcomes might differ depending on several variables, including those considered in the present study, which are type of IOS used, operator experience and the clinical scenario. Investigations comparing such variables might be useful in order to draw specific clinical indications for different IOS systems.

The results of the present study showed that the operator experience significantly affects trueness in the three analyzed clinical conditions and the null hypothesis was, therefore, rejected. However, in the single and partial rehabilitation scenarios, the experienced clinician reported better results compared to the inexperienced clinician using both IOS, suggesting that a learning curve can improve the clinical outcomes also when applying a standardized protocol for intraoral scanning. On the contrary, in the full-arch scenario, the inexperienced operator recorded better results when using OP scanner, while trueness was greater for the experienced clinician when using IT scanner. It is also interesting to note that differences among experienced and non-expert operators increased in the full-arch scenario, that was also the configuration with the lowest levels of trueness. Such outcomes confirm that intraoral scanning might be more challenging in case of implant-supported full-arch rehabilitations compared to partial rehabilitations.

Similar results were obtained by Canullo et al. [8], where in the full-arch impression using the CS3600 (Carestream) IOS better values of trueness were obtained by the unexperienced operator.

Comparing the present outcomes with those of the previously published study, trueness mean values were better in the present study compared to the previous, except for the scans made by the inexperienced operator in the full-arch with IT. Globally, OP showed the best results. While considering the single and two-implants scenarios better results were obtained with the IT and OP scanner than with CS3660 and TRIOS3 (3shape).

Additionally, Ender et al. in 2019 [14] reported that IOS are more performing for single implants or portions of dental arch, rather than full-arch. At the same time, the results seem to suggest that some IOS perform better than others in the full-arch scenario. This is confirmed by the study by Treesh et al. of 2018 [15] reporting that in full-arch rehabilitations, the accuracy of the scans depends on the type of scanner used.

Some limits of the present research must be acknowledged. First of all, this is an in vitro study and additional difficulties that are present in the mouth were not simulated (saliva, presence of the tongue, etc.) and for this reason, the results must be taken with caution. Additionally, the use of full gypsum casts instead of using the conventional casts with pink artificial gingiva it can be a confounding factor in the algorithm capture for the intra-oral scanner. On the other hand, this in vitro protocol improves the standardization of the tests, with all the digital impression made always in the same conditions, in a repeatable and comparable way.

5. Conclusions

While the experience of the operator significantly affects trueness of intraoral scanners, the outcomes of the present study suggest that obtainment of optimal trueness might be more challenging in full-arch rehabilitations compared to single and partial rehabilitations. A statistically significant difference was present among IOS in the two-implant and full-arch scenarios.

Author Contributions: Conceptualization, P.P., L.C. and M.M.; methodology, L.C., E.B. and M.A.; software, M.C.; formal analysis, N.P. and F.B.; resources, F.P.; writing—original draft preparation, N.P.; writing—review and editing, P.P. and M.M. All authors have read and agreed to the published version of the manuscript.

Funding: This research received no external funding.

Institutional Review Board Statement: Not applicable.

Informed Consent Statement: Not applicable.

Data Availability Statement: Data available on request.

Conflicts of Interest: The authors declare no conflict of interest.

References

1. Pera, F.; Pesce, P.; Bevilacqua, M.; Setti, P.; Menini, M. Analysis of Different Impression Techniques and Materials on Multiple Implants through 3-Dimensional Laser Scanner. *Implant. Dent.* **2016**, *25*, 232–237. [CrossRef] [PubMed]
2. Mormann, W.H.; Bindl, A. The new creativity in ceramic restorations: Dental CAD-CIM. *Quintessence Int.* **1996**, *27*, 821–828. [PubMed]
3. Pesce, P.; Pera, F.; Setti, P.; Menini, M. Precision and Accuracy of a Digital Impression Scanner in Full-Arch Implant Rehabilitation. *Int. J. Prosthodont.* **2018**, *31*, 171–175. [CrossRef] [PubMed]
4. Mangano, F.; Gandolfi, A.; Luongo, G.; Logozzo, S. Intraoral scanners in dentistry: A review of the current literature. *BMC Oral. Health* **2017**, *17*, 149. [CrossRef] [PubMed]
5. Gjelvold, B.; Chrcanovic, B.R.; Korduner, E.K.; Collin-Bagewitz, I.; Kisch, J. Intraoral Digital Impression Technique Compared to Conventional Impression Technique. A Randomized Clinical Trial. *J. Prosthodont.* **2016**, *25*, 282–287. [CrossRef] [PubMed]
6. Ting-Shu, S.; Jian, S. Intraoral Digital Impression Technique: A Review. *J. Prosthodont.* **2015**, *24*, 313–321. [CrossRef] [PubMed]
7. Vecsei, B.; Joos-Kovacs, G.; Borbely, J.; Hermann, P. Comparison of the accuracy of direct and indirect three-dimensional digitizing processes for CAD/CAM systems—An in vitro study. *J. Prosthodont. Res.* **2017**, *61*, 177–184. [CrossRef] [PubMed]

8. Canullo, L.; Colombo, M.; Menini, M.; Sorge, P.; Pesce, P. Trueness of Intraoral Scanners Considering Operator Experience and Three Different Implant Scenarios: A Preliminary Report. *Int. J. Prosthodont.* **2021**, *34*, 250–253. [CrossRef] [PubMed]
9. Menini, M.; Setti, P.; Pera, F.; Pera, P.; Pesce, P. Accuracy of multi-unit implant impression: Traditional techniques versus a digital procedure. *Clin. Oral. Investig.* **2018**, *22*, 1253–1262. [CrossRef] [PubMed]
10. Ahlholm, P.; Sipila, K.; Vallittu, P.; Jakonen, M.; Kotiranta, U. Digital Versus Conventional Impressions in Fixed Prosthodontics: A Review. *J. Prosthodont.* **2018**, *27*, 35–41. [CrossRef] [PubMed]
11. Zimmermann, M.; Mehl, A.; Mormann, W.H.; Reich, S. Intraoral scanning systems-a current overview. *Int. J. Comput. Dent.* **2015**, *18*, 101–129. [PubMed]
12. Ender, A.; Attin, T.; Mehl, A. In vivo precision of conventional and digital methods of obtaining complete-arch dental impressions. *J. Prosthet. Dent.* **2016**, *115*, 313–320. [CrossRef] [PubMed]
13. Guth, J.F.; Runkel, C.; Beuer, F.; Stimmelmayr, M.; Edelhoff, D.; Keul, C. Accuracy of five intraoral scanners compared to indirect digitalization. *Clin. Oral. Investig.* **2017**, *21*, 1445–1455. [CrossRef] [PubMed]
14. Ender, A.; Zimmermann, M.; Mehl, A. Accuracy of complete- and partial-arch impressions of actual intraoral scanning systems in vitro. *Int. J. Comput. Dent.* **2019**, *22*, 11–19. [PubMed]
15. Treesh, J.C.; Liacouras, P.C.; Taft, R.M.; Brooks, D.I.; Raiciulescu, S.; Ellert, D.O.; Grant, G.T.; Ye, L. Complete-arch accuracy of intraoral scanners. *J. Prosthet. Dent.* **2018**, *120*, 382–388. [CrossRef] [PubMed]

MDPI
St. Alban-Anlage 66
4052 Basel
Switzerland
Tel. +41 61 683 77 34
Fax +41 61 302 89 18
www.mdpi.com

Journal of Clinical Medicine Editorial Office
E-mail: jcm@mdpi.com
www.mdpi.com/journal/jcm

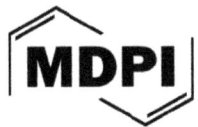

www.ingramcontent.com/pod-product-compliance
Lightning Source LLC
LaVergne TN
LVHW070606100526
838202LV00012B/578